HASHIMOTO'S PROTOCOL

A 90-Day Plan for
Reversing Thyroid Symptoms
and Getting Your Life Back

IZABELLA WENTZ
PharmD, FASCP

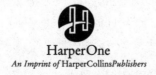

HarperOne
An Imprint of HarperCollins*Publishers*

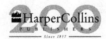

This book contains advice and information relating to health care. It should be used to supplement rather than replace the advice of your doctor or another trained health professional. If you know or suspect you have a health problem, it is recommended that you seek your physician's advice before embarking on any medical program or treatment. All efforts have been made to assure the accuracy of the information contained in this book as of the date of publication. The publisher and the author disclaim liability for any medical outcomes that may occur as a result of applying the methods suggested in this book.

HarperCollins books may be purchased for educational, business, or sales promotional use. For information, please email the Special Markets Department at SPsales@harpercollins.com.

FIRST EDITION

Designed by Indigo Editing & Publications.

Library of Congress Cataloging-in-Publication Data
Names: Wentz, Izabella, author.
Title: Hashimoto's protocol : a 90-day plan for reversing thyroid symptoms and getting your life back / Izabella Wentz, PharmD, FASCP.
Description: First edition. | New York, NY : HarperOne, [2017] | Includes bibliographical references and index.
Identifiers: LCCN 2017013622| ISBN 9780062571298 (hardback) | ISBN 9780062571311 (paperback) | ISBN 9780062660596 (audio)
Subjects: LCSH: Autoimmune thyroiditis—Popular works. | Autoimmune thyroiditis—Treatment. | Hypothyroidism—Popular works. | Hypothyroidism—Treatment. | BISAC: HEALTH & FITNESS / Diseases / Immune System. | HEALTH & FITNESS / Healing.
Classification: LCC RC657.5.T48 W45 2017 | DDC 616.4/4079—dc23 LC record available at https://lccn.loc.gov/2017013622

18 19 20 21 LSC 20 19 18 17 16 15 14 13 12

*To my dear readers, health seekers, and Root Cause Rebels,
may you recover your health so that you can follow your dreams and be
the change you want to see in this world!*

Contents

A Note to the Reader   vii

Foreword   ix

Introduction   1

Part I: Getting to Know Hashimoto's and the Root Cause Approach   13

1. My Hashimoto's Success Story—and How to Create Your Own   15
2. Understanding the Symptoms, Diagnosis, and Origins of Hashimoto's   41
3. How the Root Cause Approach Can Help You Recover Your Health   65

Part II: The Fundamental Protocols   81

4. Liver Support Protocol   83
5. Adrenal Recovery Protocol   147
6. Gut Balance Protocol   191
7. Advanced Root Cause Assessments   221

Part III: The Advanced Protocols   229

8. Protocols for Optimizing Thyroid Hormones   231
9. Protocols for Mastering Nutrition and Nutrients   259
10. Protocols for Overcoming Traumatic Stress   283
11. Protocols for Addressing Infections   307
12. Protocols for Removing Toxins   331

Author's Note   355

Gratitude   357

Selected Bibliography   359

Index   365

A Note to the Reader

Dear Reader,

If you've picked up this book, chances are that you are struggling with your personal health and you know or suspect it has something to do with your thyroid. Maybe you just learned that you have the autoimmune condition Hashimoto's thyroiditis and you're looking for answers on how to get your health back. Or perhaps you've been taking thyroid medications for years and have heard that there may be another path to feeling better—and now you're ready to take it.

For many, you have arrived here as a result of a growing list of confusing symptoms with possible origins in thyroid dysfunction. These could include experiencing hair loss, anxiety, joint pain, gastrointestinal distress, extreme fatigue, allergies, and acid reflux (to name just a few of the potential symptoms).

Whatever your story with Hashimoto's, you've come to the right place, and I'm here to help. I experienced symptoms of Hashimoto's for over a decade, and I chased a diagnosis for many of those years. I understand the frustration that comes with the lack of answers and the lack of support from the conventional medical paradigm. I also know what it's like to feel like you need to figure everything out on your own.

It was only after I applied my pharmacist's training, dedicated thousands of hours to research, and became my own human guinea pig that I was able to produce a protocol for healing. I was able to get my health back and have now guided thousands of others to improved health and in turn a happier and more fulfilling life.

Wherever you are in your journey, I want you to know that things can get better, and you will get better, as long as you commit to take charge of your own health and make changes in your life. Getting this book is an excellent first step, and I'm so happy that you picked up *Hashimoto's Protocol: A 90-Day Plan for Reversing Thyroid Symptoms and Getting Your Life Back.* I'm honored to be a part of your journey!

Izabella Wentz, PharmD, FASCP

Foreword

The guiding principle of *Hashimoto's Protocol*, "Genes are not your destiny!" is something I truly believe in. I tell my patients that genetics load the gun, but environment pulls the trigger. The way you eat, how much you exercise, how you manage stress, and your exposure to environmental toxins all contribute to the formation and progression of chronic disease.

Over 133 million Americans suffer from chronic disease, with an estimated 20 million Americans living with some form of thyroid disease. The symptoms of Hashimoto's and hypothyroidism go well beyond low energy and can have a catastrophic impact on your health. The thyroid gland determines the speed of, and enhances the activity of, every function in your body. It determines your mood, skin and hair health, heart function, blood sugar levels, fertility, body temperature, muscle function, and hormonal function especially with symptoms related to PMS and menopause.

When Izabella Wentz, PharmD, was first diagnosed with Hashimoto's, she quickly discovered there was a significant lack of knowledge about lifestyle interventions for Hashimoto's. Faced with her own illness, she methodically researched and tested healing protocols to achieve her personal remission. Then she bravely shared her process with the world, leading the way for other Hashimoto's patients to follow in her footsteps. Not only have thousands of patients read and successfully applied the research from her first book, *Hashimoto's Thyroiditis: Lifestyle Interventions for Finding and Treating the Root Cause,* but she has also been a strong voice in the medical world in building awareness about Hashimoto's and championing the functional medicine approach.

As a strong advocate of functional medicine, which addresses the root cause of disease, not just the symptoms, I am an admirer of Dr. Wentz's Fundamental Protocol approach, which will help you get to the root of your illness by focusing on three key areas.

First, Dr. Wentz's Liver Support Protocol will give you the steps to reduce your toxic burden, support your body's own detoxification pathways, and make you more resilient against the chemical warfare in our environment. Environmental toxins can feed thyroid dysfunction and related health conditions through inflammation, oxidative stress, and mitochondrial injury. Our environment affects our genes. The genetic code itself may not change, but the world around us highly influences the way those genes are expressed. Our environment has changed more in the last one hundred years than in all of previous human history. The Liver Support Protocol shows you how to take action. Wentz walks you through removing toxins from your home and food supply all while supporting your natural detoxification pathways by adding in superfoods, activities, and supplements to lower your body's toxic burden.

Second, the Adrenal Recovery Protocol will give you the steps to improve your thyroid function through adrenal balance. As a functional medicine doctor, I know that any patient with poor thyroid function must address the effects of chronic stress and provide support to the adrenal glands as part of the healing process. Wentz teaches you how to boost your stress resilience through her Adrenal Recovery Protocol, which guides patients through the restorative steps of resting, reducing stress and inflammation, balancing blood sugar, and replenishing key nutrients.

Lastly, the Gut Balance Protocol provides Hashimoto's patients with the tools they need to heal intestinal permeability and regain optimal health. Patients living with irritable bowel syndrome or leaky gut often struggle with debilitating symptoms like bloating, stomach pain, diarrhea, and constipation. Wentz suggests strategies in line with those I've found to eliminate irritable bowel syndrome symptoms and restore healthy gut function in most of my patients, including removing reactive foods, balancing gut flora, and supplementing with enzymes and nutrients to nourish the gut.

I'm also excited about the innovative research shared in the Advanced Protocols, which will allow patients to halt the progression of autoimmunity by identifying and removing triggers and not just optimize their thyroid hormone levels through the use of appropriate medications but also reverse the autoimmune thyroid damage sustained, allowing many patients to taper their medications under their doctor's supervision and to live their life to the fullest.

Hashimoto's Protocol provides the opportunity to change the way both patients and doctors think about Hashimoto's treatment and recovery. By using a broad approach that deals with the underlying cause of disease and not simply subduing symptoms, Wentz has paved the way for you to return to health in the most pragmatic time frame possible. This book provides you with the opportunity to take charge of your own health by supporting you with the tools and knowledge necessary to put your healing into action!

Dr. Wentz reminds patients that with the guidance of a functional medicine doctor, patients can take a proactive approach to correcting their thyroid issues and putting their autoimmune condition into remission.

Mark Hyman, MD
Ten-time #1 *New York Times* bestselling author
Director, Cleveland Clinic Center for Functional Medicine
Founder and Director, The UltraWellness Center

Introduction

While Hashimoto's thyroiditis certainly sounds like a rare and exotic disorder, the fact is that Hashimoto's is the most common autoimmune condition in the United States and worldwide, affecting anywhere from 13.4 percent to 38 percent of people within the general population. Synthetic thyroid hormones have topped the national drug bestseller lists for the last three years, and most individuals taking thyroid hormones have Hashimoto's.

The rate of Hashimoto's is increasing with every passing decade. Conservative estimates state that *one in five* women will be affected with Hashimoto's or another thyroid disorder at some point in their lives. Many individuals who have this condition may not be aware that they have it, whether it's because they haven't been properly tested or because they've only been told that they have a "sluggish" or "underactive" thyroid (when really they have Hashimoto's). All this is to say that if you have Hashimoto's or suspect that you do, you are certainly not a lone soul in the crowd.

If you have Hashimoto's, the immune system recognizes the thyroid gland as a foreign invader and launches an immune response against it as if it were an invading virus, bacteria, or other pathogen. This autoimmune destruction of the thyroid gland eventually results in the thyroid no longer being able to produce sufficient thyroid hormone. This in turn leads to a hypothyroid condition.

Do You Have Hashimoto's, Hypothyroidism, or Both?

Hypothyroidism, by definition, is a clinical state of low levels of thyroid hormone in the body. The low levels of thyroid hormone can occur as a result of a variety of different reasons, such as iodine deficiency, surgical removal of the thyroid gland, excess use of thyroid-suppressing medications, pituitary suppression, or damage to the thyroid (physical or disease induced).

Hashimoto's causes most cases of hypothyroidism in the United States, Canada, Europe, and in other countries that add iodine to their salt supply. Depending on the source, estimates are that between 90 and 97 percent of those diagnosed with hypothyroidism in the United States actually have Hashimoto's.

Despite Hashimoto's being the underlying cause for hypothyroidism, after being diagnosed, many people are told that their thyroid is "underactive," "sluggish," or that they *"just have hypothyroidism."* However, very few are told *why* their thyroid is no longer producing enough hormones or that they have an autoimmune condition. What they are usually told is that they'll be just fine as long as they remember to take their synthetic thyroid medications each morning for the rest of their lives. Most patients never think to ask the question, "Why is my immune system attacking my thyroid?" Therefore they never know to address the immune system imbalance and never get an opportunity to prevent or reverse the progression of the disease. The doctor is simply treating the symptoms, and the patient is doing exactly what we have all been trained to do: take the expert advice and try to move on with our lives. There is another way.

Many doctors simply don't test their patients for Hashimoto's. That's because the conventional medical model treats autoimmune thyroid disorders in the same way as it would treat someone with a nutrient-deficiency-induced thyroid disorder, someone with a congenital defect of the thyroid gland, someone who was born without a thyroid, or someone who had their thyroid removed or treated

At-Risk Populations

Hashimoto's runs in families, is five to eight times more common in women, and tends to peak around puberty, pregnancy, and perimenopause. If you've been diagnosed with Hashimoto's, I would encourage you to urge your daughters, sisters, mothers, aunts, and grandmothers to get tested, especially if they are in the age range of these three most common times for thyroid hormone abnormalities to surface. Also, just because the condition is more common in women does not mean that men or children are not affected.

with radioactive iodine. Conventional medicine treats all of these conditions with synthetic thyroid hormones. But for all of those who suffer with Hashimoto's, this is a life-altering mistake.

My Experience with Hashimoto's

My journey with Hashimoto's thyroiditis began in 2009 when I was diagnosed with the condition. I knew about the disease because we'd covered thyroid disorders in pharmacy school, but at the time I hadn't paid the topic any special attention. We had one short lecture in which I learned about some of the symptoms of thyroid hormone imbalances. The lecture also made a point that women were more likely to become hypothyroid as they became older and that the treatment of choice was synthetic thyroid hormone. The lecture did note that most cases of hypothyroidism were autoimmune, due to Hashimoto's, but besides that, my lecture notes were devoid of any substantial information (and I always took really great notes!).

My interest in Hashimoto's was prompted by my own diagnosis, which came when I was just twenty-seven, obviously throwing my understanding of Hashimoto's as a disease of aging out the window. The diagnosis had not come easily. I had spent almost a decade visiting doctors with my strange symptoms before I was finally diagnosed (I'll go into my story in greater detail in chapter 1). Even after receiving my diagnosis, the help offered by my well-meaning conventional doctors seemed shortsighted. The only recommendation by my doctor was a prescription medication to replace the hormones my thyroid was no longer able to make, as my own thyroid was under attack by the immune system. It felt like pouring more water into a leaky bucket. My logic told me, why not try to stop the attack on the thyroid? I knew there had to be a better way. So I decided to take on overcoming Hashimoto's as a personal life mission, the first step being to design my own protocol to heal myself.

Ultimately, a protocol that incorporated specific dietary changes, strategic supplements, and innovative medications to address the underlying root causes of my condition was what started to make me feel better and eventually led to remission in January of 2013.

Throughout the process, I had kept a detailed journal in which I noted my research and progress. And these notes became the beginning of my first book, *Hashimoto's Thyroiditis: Lifestyle Interventions for Finding and Treating the Root Cause*. Based on the book's success—it became a *New York Times* bestseller—it became clear to me that there was an audience looking for solutions to Hashimoto's just as I had been.

I began providing consultations for people with Hashimoto's and their treating clinicians. And since that time, I've collected over five hundred success stories from readers, clients, and health care professionals who were also able to see tremendous improvements in their symptoms, autoimmune thyroid markers, and labs when they used the strategies I recommended.

I've had the pleasure of meeting the brightest minds in functional medicine and natural health, and I have had fascinating discussions about innovative treatment strategies. Having worked with over a

The DIG-AT-IT Approach

In my first book, I introduced the DIG-AT-IT approach to identifying the triggers associated with Hashimoto's. The acronym DIG-AT-IT stands for:

Depletions, Digestion
Iodine, Inflammation, Infection, Immune Imbalance
Gut, Gluten
Adrenals, Alkaline Phosphatase
Triggers
Intolerances
Toxins

thousand people with Hashimoto's, I developed a streamlined approach to help people strengthen their bodies and walk them through the maze of identifying their individual triggers to autoimmune thyroid disease.

Helping individuals with Hashimoto's has become not just my passion but also my full-time job and life calling. In addition to my client work, I'm also an ardent advocate of spreading awareness about recovering from Hashimoto's, and I run a website, Facebook community, and popular newsletter dedicated to sharing innovative strategies on overcoming Hashimoto's. To date, I've surveyed my community of over 250,000 Root Cause Rebels as to the interventions that have helped them the most.

While I don't have all the answers to solving Hashimoto's, I've had a tremendous amount of success with helping myself and guiding others with Hashimoto's to improved health, reduced symptoms, and in some cases, elimination of the autoimmune attack on the body as well as the need for medications.

Can Hashimoto's Be Cured?

While there is no cure for Hashimoto's, in this book I'm going to give you detailed information on how the condition can be reversed in as little as ninety days.

I'm talking about eliminating all of your symptoms, restoring your energy levels, getting you on target to a healthy weight, growing your hair back, and helping you feel alive again. You'll learn about the potential triggers that have led you to develop Hashimoto's and how to eliminate them. You'll learn how to replenish your nutrients and your levels of thyroid hormone, and you'll learn how to stop the autoimmune attacks on your body.

Many of you will be able to see a reduction in your autoimmune markers, and some of you may no longer test positive for Hashimoto's once you implement the recommendations in this book. A small subset of you may even be able to regenerate thyroid tissue and discontinue thyroid medications (under your doctor's supervision).

Scientists have said that there is no cure for Hashimoto's, but I believe we have the capacity and knowledge to put the condition into remission for most people. Each autoimmune condition has a different definition of what remission may mean. To me, I like to think of remission as a journey, not necessarily a destination. Here are the scenic stopping points of the remission journey:

- Feeling better
- Eliminating all of your symptoms
- Reducing your thyroid antibodies
  - First under 100 IU/mL
  - Then under 35 IU/mL
- Regenerating thyroid tissue
- Experiencing a functional cure

Healing from Hashimoto's should be a stepwise approach, and if you are feeling unwell, your first focus will likely be to start feeling better! In many cases, this means getting on the right type of thyroid hormones, at the right dose.

Once you've been able to eliminate your symptoms, reduce your thyroid antibodies to the range of a person without disease (<35 IU/mL), and regenerate thyroid tissue, will you still have Hashimoto's? To answer this, we have to consider the origins of autoimmune disease. Recent medical advances have determined that three factors are necessary for autoimmunity to develop:

- The genetic predisposition
- Triggers that turn on the genes
- Intestinal permeability

Obviously we can't change our genes, but we can address our triggers and intestinal permeability. What's even more exciting is that we can turn off gene expression by eliminating triggers and intestinal permeability, leading to remission.

We no longer manifest the symptoms of the condition, and we no longer have an autoimmune response to our thyroid. In some people, thyroid function returns spontaneously, while in others, thanks to new innovative approaches outlined in chapter 8, we now have the means to restore thyroid function in up to 50 percent of those with Hashimoto's.

At that point, once we are asymptomatic, there is no longer an autoimmune reaction to the thyroid gland, and our own thyroid is producing thyroid hormones without the need for thyroid medications, we can say that we've reached a functional cure. Once here, we will no longer show any signs or symptoms of the condition.

Some will argue that you will still have Hashimoto's, and genetically speaking, this is true. You will be at risk for developing the condition again, especially if you come across specific environmental triggers, which current research shows can turn on our gene expression. Repeat exposure to the triggers may switch on your

Hashimoto's-producing genes and reignite the autoimmune attack on the thyroid. But genes are not our destiny.

Conventional medical doctors will insist that there is no way to reduce the attack on your own thyroid gland, but my experiences—both my own and with patients—as well as the experiences of numerous functional and integrative clinicians in my network, have shown this isn't the case.

At the time of my Hashimoto's diagnosis, I struggled with chronic fatigue, weight gain, hair loss, irritable bowel syndrome, carpal tunnel, joint pain, acid reflux, brain fog, a chronic cough, multiple allergies, bloating, anxiety, palpitations, pale skin, cold intolerance, acne, and much more. I'm happy to report that one by one, all my symptoms have disappeared. I spend most of my days with a head full of hair, ideas, and quick-wittedness. I'm happy, fit, calm, and energetic, and I can finally pursue my life passions.

Oftentimes, experts will say that once you have Hashimoto's, you'll always have Hashimoto's, but this is like saying that someone who had a urinary tract infection will always have a urinary tract infection. Urinary tract infections are treatable, and of course you can always get another one, if you are infected with bacteria again. Having a urinary tract and being a woman puts us at risk for getting urinary tract infections, just as having a thyroid gland and the genetic predisposition to develop autoimmune thyroid disease puts us at risk for developing Hashimoto's.

Of course, just as we can take precautions to prevent urinary tract infections—like acidifying our urine, using certain preventive supplements like D-mannose or cranberry extract, practicing proper urinary hygiene, and using biofilm-busting enzymes to break down colonies of urinary bacteria that promote chronic, recurrent urinary infections—we can also use targeted strategies for preventing flare-ups of Hashimoto's. Remember, genes are not our destiny. The Root Cause Approach interventions I recommend in this book will teach you not just about trigger avoidance but also about how to become more resilient.

Why My Approach Is Different

While the health care model relies on people being sick (after all, that's what keeps us coming back to clinics and pharmacies month after month), my goal is to show you how you can feel better through lifestyle choices and by addressing the root cause of your condition so you can reduce your dependence on the medical system. Because after all, while medications can treat a disease, lifestyle interventions are the real path to lifelong wellness.

My deepest desire for my first book was that it would give people hope and tools to recover their health, and I'm thrilled to have received numerous success stories of people who were able to feel better, get their health back, and go into remission after reading the book.

The decision to write the book you're reading was made after I met Teresa, one of my wonderful readers, at a lecture I gave in Chicago back in 2014. Teresa had seen a tremendous amount of improvement in her own health after reading *Hashimoto's Thyroiditis*, but she had a special request for me:

> I am so grateful for your book, and I love digging for my own health. But it would save me so much time and it would be so much easier if you could just give me a specific protocol. Which exact supplements should I take? Have you considered making supplements specifically for people with Hashimoto's? Can you tell me what exactly I should eat and not eat?

Teresa's request reflected those expressed by many of my other readers. While some people said that they loved learning everything about Hashimoto's and how to DIG-AT-IT for their own individual root cause, many others felt overwhelmed with digging for their own health—they wanted a done-for-them, streamlined protocol. And this is how the concept of *Hashimoto's Protocol* was born.

I had previously been very careful about not recommending specific brands of supplements or specific diets and letting people make their own choices. I've always been the kind of person who likes to do her own research and wanted to give people the same courtesy. However, meeting readers like Teresa and working with clients one-on-one made me realize that while many people love to learn everything they can about the condition they have, and love to DIG-AT-IT for their own individual root causes, others felt overwhelmed by it.

Of course as a health nerd, this was a bit challenging for me to understand at first, until I took a Pilates class with a very intense instructor. This woman was brilliant and seemed to know everything about movement and human physiology, yet her knowledge was lost on me. During our first lesson, she told me all about every muscle that was worked with each movement and even gave me a folder of Pilates homework to do on my own time. But all I wanted was to look toned in my swimsuit. I didn't really care about the science behind how to get there or whether the movement I was doing was impacting my rectus abdominis or gluteus maximus. It's not like I wanted to become a Pilates expert!

I now understand why Teresa and so many others requested a plan. It became evident that to truly help as many people as possible, I needed to develop and perfect my protocol. The book in your hands comes from years of training and clinical research. It holds the latest and most up-to-date scientific research and cutting-edge treatments for Hashimoto's—this book is the culmination of my passion and life's work, and I am thrilled to share it with you.

Hashimoto's Protocol features specific protocols, success stories, and recipes that you can use to get your health back. This book is in large part created by my Hashimoto's community of Root Cause Rebels, as many of you have generously submitted your success stories with the hope that they would help other people uncover their root causes. You will see their insights and stories sprinkled throughout this book!

In addition to giving you a plan to feel better through going after individual triggers, this book will also focus on making you more resilient so you will become less susceptible to flare-ups of Hashimoto's even when you are faced with additional triggers. This book focuses on helping you achieve the following goals:

- Finally feeling better
- Reducing the autoimmune attack in your body
- Identifying your individual triggers
- Reversing your condition

For the science and health nerds who want to have a deeper understanding of the *why* behind the *what,* I will also include science sections throughout the book as well as a comprehensive protocol and testing guide that will allow you to dig deeper if you want.

I am so glad that you are here, and I'm so excited for the improvements in your health and your entire life that will come from you taking charge of your own health. So let's get started on creating your success story!

PART I

GETTING TO KNOW HASHIMOTO'S AND THE ROOT CAUSE APPROACH

My Hashimoto's Success Story— and How to Create Your Own

When I was diagnosed with Hashimoto's in 2009, I was working as a consultant pharmacist for a case management agency in Southern California. The agency was dedicated to helping people with disabilities live the most fulfilling lives they could live.

I was part of a team that included physicians, nurses, psychologists, case managers, and often a behaviorist or psychiatrist. The role of our team was to figure out if there were underlying medical, situational, behavioral, pharmacological, or psychological issues that were contributing to our clients' health concerns.

Most of the clients were not able to articulate what was going on with them due to their disabilities, so oftentimes the only way we knew that they were in pain was when they became aggressive, had vocal outbursts, or were uncooperative. I was the sole pharmacist on the team and performed case reviews for thousands of clients in my time with the agency.

While my official job title was Consultant Pharmacist, I really felt that the most important part of my job was to help advocate for individuals with disabilities who could not voice their health concerns. I ensured that they were getting the most benefit from their medications, that they were not overmedicated, that they had access to medications that could potentially help them, and that they received the proper care they deserved.

Many of my clients had been placed on heavy-duty psychotropic medications when their caregivers deemed them uncooperative, aggressive, or loud. Our job was to prevent this from happening.

I loved my job and was excited to start my workday every morning. Advocating for others who were suffering in silence had fulfilled my lifelong goal of helping people, yet like my clients, I too was suffering in my own way.

I had embarrassing problems that I did not want to share with anyone else in my life: acid reflux that manifested as a chronic cough at the worst possible times (during client meetings, presentations, and so on), irritable bowel syndrome (IBS) that made the bathroom my "second office," terrible anxiety that made me break into a cold sweat when it was my turn to speak up in team meetings and jump out of my seat every time someone knocked on my office door, constant leg cramping, and muscle pains. To top it all off, I had carpal tunnel in both hands that shot up my arms and was so bad that I needed to wear arm braces to perform my job functions and eventually had to use dictation software for all of my emails and reports.

Additionally, my forty-hour workweek and commute were leaving me exhausted. I had dreams of going dancing with my husband, meeting friends in Los Angeles hot spots, learning a new language, and writing in my spare time, but all I could do when I got home was eat, watch TV, and fall asleep on the couch.

I couldn't grasp how our disabled clients were able to go to day programs or jobs for forty hours each week. Here I was an "able-bodied" young woman who needed to go to bed by 9:00 P.M. every night just so I could wake up at 8:00 A.M. to start my nine-to-five job.

And of course, I looked fine. Though I felt bloated and out of shape, I technically wasn't overweight or underweight, and I didn't need crutches to walk. I had hair on my head, and I didn't have visible scars, rashes, or bandages that would make people think I was in pain.

Working with people with disabilities made me appreciate the health I did have, but at the same time, my compassion for them made me minimize my own suffering. I had always been a person who put everyone else's needs before my own, so naturally I was drawn to the healing professions, but sadly my care for others led me to put off my own care.

As much as I tried to ignore my own health problems, the fact was, I was in pain every day and this was beginning to interfere with the job I loved, my ability to be the wife I wanted to be, and my life-long dream of creating positive change in the world.

My symptoms only increased. I became allergic to everything, including my sweet dog and all of the native trees and bushes in California. I was cold all of the time. I found myself taking numerous medications—cough suppressants, acid reflux medications, nonsteroi-dal anti-inflammatory drugs (NSAIDs), and allergy medications—which of course came with numerous side effects!

Worst of all, I was losing my memory. In high school, college, and grad school, I would joke that I just had to look at a piece of paper to remember everything that was on it. I was always super sharp and quick, and I had the ability to remember details of conversations that had taken place years before.

But now I had terrible brain fog. I would walk into rooms and forget why. I would lose common words midsentence ("You know, that animal with the fur? Yes, a cat!"). It was a really scary feeling, and it got so bad that I took an assessment to rule out dementia. It was also exhausting trying to hide my embarrassing memory problems from the people in my life. I thought I was doing a good job at hiding them until one day when my husband made a comment, "Well, honey, I know how your memory is, so I've decided to write things out for you so you can look at them later." I was devastated. I felt like I was losing myself and my mind, and now other people were noticing.

"Well, You're Just Getting Older ..."

I went to numerous doctors with the hope of receiving some answers, but most of them told me that all the symptoms I was experiencing were "normal," "not a big deal," and some suggested, "Perhaps they're just in your head." I was prescribed medications for allergies, acid reflux, and even an antidepressant for my "anxiety."

One of the most amusing answers I got was "Well, you're just getting older. We tend to lose our memory, get more tired, and put on weight when we get older." Did I mention I was twenty-six at the time?

Through all of this, I thought of myself as a good role model of health. I hardly ever went out to eat and made most of my meals from scratch, opting for whole wheat, low-fat dairy, and minimal red meat. I often brought home-cooked quiches and baked muffins and pies to share with my coworkers, and I loved baking whole-grain cookies for my husband and even special whole wheat treats for our dog.

I tried so hard to be healthy. I would meet coworkers during lunch to walk or do workout videos, and I often hit the gym on my way home from work (but all of this made me more tired). I did not smoke and limited my drinking to rare social occasions. I was too tired to do anything social, though, since the demands of day-to-day life like running errands and cleaning my house left me exhausted!

I began to think this was my life and I just had to accept it. I had grown accustomed to my IBS, bloating, and fatigue. I had grown accustomed to waking up, going to work, coming home, eating, and sleeping without having the energy to pursue my dreams of traveling, writing, connecting with people, taking courses, and changing the world.

By the time I was twenty-seven, my symptoms had been with me for almost a decade and had been steadily getting worse. What started as minor symptoms that would come and go with minimal effect on my day-to-day life had now become life altering. I had given up on doctors—most of them told me that I was either depressed, stressed, or suffering from IBS and that I just had to learn to live with all of the symptoms I was having. Others said that all the symptoms were in my head. I knew I wasn't depressed, but I realized maybe it was time to just accept that the IBS, chronic fatigue, memory loss, and other mystery conditions were just part of my fate. I stopped seeking help and suffered in silence.

Then, things got so much worse. I began to have panic attacks. My husband would go out jogging, and if more than fifteen minutes passed, I would get into my car to start looking for him, fearing that he'd gotten into an accident or, even worse, that he had met another woman and ran off with her! Of course, I knew I wasn't being rational, but I couldn't help freaking out.

My hair lost its luster and started falling out in clumps (this was very difficult for a Leo who liked to check out her mane every time she passed a mirror). My skin started to look really dry, and I began to have wrinkles and puffy eyes, and my face always seemed to look bloated. I was in my twenties and supposed to be in my prime, but I felt old and tired.

I seemed to have become allergic to everything, and my chronic cough woke me up throughout the night and drove me crazy. I had to wear my carpal tunnel braces 24-7 and stop doing yoga, my favorite hobby, entirely. I had to cut back on client case reviews, which required a lot of writing and documentation. These had always been my favorite part of my job, because I got to meet with my clients face-to-face and complete a comprehensive review of their health needs.

Eventually, I'd had enough. I was a newlywed and felt like my health and life were falling apart. My new husband and family members wondered why I seemed to be getting worse and worse. The chronic cough drove me crazy. I remember confiding in my colleague, "I'm just about ready to cut off my head if it means the cough would stop." I began to desperately search for answers.

Can you relate?

I decided to go "doctor shopping" again, but this time I had become more skilled at navigating the system. My time as a consultant pharmacist and patient advocate had made me aware of the fact that doctors—while most of the time are very well-meaning—did not know everything about my body. I was going to need to advocate for myself in order to get to the bottom of my health condition.

I went to various doctors and asked for diagnostic tests, looking for answers based on my symptoms. Some of the doctors were extremely caring and sympathetic, others completely dismissive, but I wasn't deterred and didn't stop until I got an answer.

A Diagnosis at Last

Eventually, I learned that I had the autoimmune condition Hashimoto's thyroiditis, which had resulted in subclinical hypothyroidism, also known as mild thyroid gland failure. I finally had a reason for my hair loss, emotional imbalance, anxiety, fatigue, and most of my other symptoms. A part of me was relieved to have a diagnosis, but I was also very disappointed. I was a young health care professional, trying my best to be healthy, and yet my body was betraying me. After all, according to conventional medical knowledge, it was my own body attacking itself, not some mystery bug, and there was nothing that could be done to stop the attack.

The initial weeks were full of grief. I cried to my husband, mom, and best friend, expressing my worries that I would never feel better, be able to have children, or feel pretty ever again (I had lost over a third of my hair and ended up dyeing it blond and getting a bob cut to cover up the in-between hair spots, but they still seemed really visible to me).

But then I woke up one day and thought about my clients. If they could be happy with all of their limitations and keep going, then I too could do the same. I decided that if I was going to be a person with Hashimoto's, I would be the healthiest person possible with Hashimoto's.

At the time, I spent a lot of time on the PubMed website, which holds the largest database of clinical trials and medical research articles. Many of my clients had rare disorders that did not have a well-defined best-practice medical approach, and this often meant that the only place to get helpful information was through case studies and research articles. I used the same methodology to find what was out there on Hashimoto's and autoimmune disease.

I also began visiting patient discussion forums, as patients would often be the first to report positive and negative experiences with various treatments for conditions. I knew firsthand that patients always had the most valuable insights, sometimes several years before the information became accepted as a medical fact.

With appreciation for the patient experience of a condition, I began to do my research into Hashimoto's. Between PubMed and patient forums, I was hoping to find information about innovative treatment options as well as lifestyle interventions. During pharmacy school, my professors had always stressed that when it came to chronic conditions, lifestyle interventions should be used before medication in mild cases and alongside medication in advanced cases. This was the approach I used once I became a consultant pharmacist as well. My team always asked about lifestyle before we considered a prescription.

In cases of depression: before prescribing selective serotonin reuptake inhibitors (SSRIs), we'd ask, how about counseling and therapy? If a person was already on medications, would they benefit from psychotherapy? In type 2 diabetes: before prescribing metformin, we'd ask, did the person have a nutritional consult?

You get the idea. Just about every common condition had a lifestyle recommendation … but at the time I couldn't find any lifestyle recommendations for Hashimoto's and autoimmune disease. I even tried turning to my trusted medical books and texts on the subject, but they were no help. Neither were any of my colleagues, my doctors, not even the endocrinologist I consulted.

The response I got from most doctors was, "If you have hypothyroidism due to Hashimoto's, take synthetic thyroid hormones to replace the hormones your body is no longer making. Then, as your

Root Cause Reflection: Sometimes It's the Patient Who Knows Best

During 2006, when I was working as a community pharmacist, one of my patients reported that the generic version of the antidepressant Wellbutrin didn't work as well as the branded version of the drug. I exchanged the drug for the branded version and filed a report with the Food and Drug Administration (FDA). Two more patients came forward with the same concern that month, and I filed an FDA report each time.

It wasn't until three years later in 2009 that this information made it to the clinical databases, and it didn't reach mainstream until October 2012, when the FDA finally decided to recall the generic drug.

This means that it took the mainstream medical world almost six years (!) to admit to a simple issue that one of my own patients had realized within just a few days of taking the medication. This is just one small example. It takes time to create change in a system as big as our medical system.

What are some things you have noticed about your health that have been ignored by the mainstream medical system?

own thyroid becomes more damaged, we will increase your dose. Since you're now at a greater risk for other autoimmune diseases, we'll also monitor you for these. With one autoimmune condition, the chances of developing another one will increase."

While these were very well-meaning individuals (some of them were my dear friends and colleagues), there was a huge gap in lifestyle knowledge for Hashimoto's. This is why I set out to change the system.

Continuing the Search for a Lifestyle Intervention

I wasn't convinced that was all there was to it. As a health consultant, I had seen firsthand that doctors certainly didn't know everything. One of many examples was a little girl with cerebral palsy who was referred to our team due to violent outbursts and screaming—her doctors wanted to give her antipsychotics, but my team found she was actually in pain and recommended physical therapy first. Within a few weeks, she was back to her previous sweet and happy demeanor. The violent outbursts had been her way of expressing her pain, and the medications would have likely just sedated her! Perhaps there was some new information out there about Hashimoto's that the average doctor and patient did not know.

I jumped into research to find a set of lifestyle interventions that could help my thyroid disorder. I quickly landed on a promising article that connected celiac disease and Hashimoto's (I wondered, *Could there be a dietary change I could make?*). I took the article to my endocrinologist appointment (I had waited almost two months before I could be seen), to make sure I was doing all that I could be doing for myself and I was heading in the right direction.

The endocrinologist I saw was very kind, but once again I was told that all I could do was take a medication to replace my thyroid hormones. He even said that most of my symptoms, including my hair loss and mood, were not related to the thyroid. And that the path was set—my immune system would continue to attack my thyroid, and I would need to increase my dosage of medications until my thyroid was completely destroyed. I would be at greater risk of developing another autoimmune condition, which could potentially be quite debilitating, like lupus or multiple sclerosis, but diet had nothing to do with it, he assured me, and there was simply nothing more I could do to make it better. He told me it wasn't my fault, which I appreciated and believed, but at the same time, it was very disempowering to be told just to wait and watch and do nothing as my immune system attacked my body.

So I went home with my prescription and cried. I thought about having lupus (we'd spent a great amount of time on it in pharmacy school), going bald, and not being able to have babies, and I felt completely hopeless.

But of course I didn't give up. I continued my search and made myself into a human guinea pig. Trying various alternative, innovative, lifestyle, and functional medicine interventions. Tracking my outcomes including subjective symptoms and objective thyroid markers like thyroid antibodies, heart rate, blood pressure, and thyroid-stimulating hormone (TSH). Hacking my own biology.

Most of 2010 was spent on trying various interventions including the immune-modulating medication low-dose naltrexone, compounded thyroid medications, dehydroepiandrosterone (DHEA), progesterone, and pregnenolone (you can learn more about my interventions in my first book, *Hashimoto's Thyroiditis*). Some of my thyroid symptoms improved after these interventions—Southern California turned out to be warm after all, and my memory and energy started to show improvements. Still, I continued to struggle with reflux, IBS, bloating, carpal tunnel, headaches, and allergies. At that point, I realized that a more holistic approach was required. I didn't just do one thing to get better—I did numerous things to get better!

In 2011, I was finally able to see remarkable improvements in my health. I made a New Year's resolution that I would do everything to get my health back. I began working with an integrative physician who encouraged me to remove gluten and dairy from my diet, and the change was remarkable. Within three days, my acid reflux, bloating, and IBS were gone. Through my own research and further guidance from other professionals, I started utilizing supplements and modifying my diet further. The carpal tunnel resolved in a few weeks, and my anxiety decreased over the course of just a few months. I was motivated to keep going.

Along the way, I had kept a detailed journal of my research notes and my progress. After all, brain fog makes it hard to remember

Welcome, Root Cause Readers

If you read my first book, I'm honored to have you here again with me, trusting me to offer you even more guidance with specific done-for-you protocols that will guide you through supporting your liver, adrenals, and gut. I hope that this book will give you the dietary guidance, supplement protocols (including specific brand recommendations), and lifestyle modifications that will address any remaining concerns and health challenges you may be facing. Like most of my Root Cause Rebels, you'll find that even if you have followed the plan in my first book, you'll benefit from the complete ninety-day protocol in the Fundamental Protocols in this book. Should your symptoms remain even after this is completed, you will want to turn to the Advanced Protocols, which will help address underlying infections, medication issues, and other unresolved triggers. I'm excited to continue to be a part of your journey!

things, so I wanted to be sure that I wasn't rereading the same information over and over again.

Ultimately, I ended up compiling a significant amount of material on how to address Hashimoto's, and it seemed too valuable to keep it just to myself. Encouraged by my mom and husband (my two biggest supporters), I decided to turn my organized notes and journals into a patient guide. My husband had already written two books detailing his experience in running ultramarathons and encouraged me to write about my own experience.

My mom, who is a physician from Poland and who has always been interested in medical advances, helped me with writing the book. She also lovingly nudged me to finish it so that we could translate it into Polish and share it with my cousins and aunts who were also diagnosed with Hashimoto's.

I was able to get into remission in January 2013, and the patient guide, *Hashimoto's Thyroiditis: Lifestyle Interventions for Finding and Treating the Root Cause*, was published on May 31 of the same year. Finally, I felt like my health struggles had a deeper purpose. Once I was able to recover my health, I was also able to turn my past challenges into my life's work, educating and empowering an increasingly large number of people to take back their health.

Now, my hope is that I can help your life turn a corner by introducing you to steps that will help reduce and hopefully eliminate your symptoms. But as much as I can try to spell it out for you, I can't *make the changes* for you—you have to put the plan into action. Things are going to get better, but the change has to come from you. Let's take a look at how you can get ready to create your own success story.

Taking Charge of Your Own Health

The first step in taking charge of your own health is to dream big and set goals. We will focus on where you are later—for now, let's focus on where you want to be. If you don't have a health journal yet, now would be a great time to start one. Journaling is one of the best ways to track your progress and any challenges and successes. If you're high tech, you may prefer to keep a journal on your computer, or if you're old school like me, you may prefer a good old-fashioned notebook. Whatever you choose, pick a journaling method you are likely to stick to. Start by reflecting on the following questions and writing down your answers:

What are your health goals?
Do you want to have more energy?
Do you want to lose that extra twenty pounds?
Do you want your hair to grow back?

The Way of the Wounded Healer

Ever since I was a little girl, I dreamed about helping other people. I became obsessed with science after learning about the scientific method in grade school, and I often pondered dedicating my life to science like Marie Curie, my idol, the first woman to win a Nobel Prize.

I became interested in pharmacology in high school and often read my mom's medical textbooks in my spare time. I wanted to find a cure for a disease so I could help others, and I decided that I would become a pharmacist. I initially thought that I would focus on mental health (I myself had experienced depression due to undiagnosed thyroid disease in my younger days) but became very discouraged after a bout of mono that left me exhausted and unable to focus on my studies.

Ever since that infection, I continued to see a decline in my health, and I often pitied myself. *Why me? Why do I have to suffer and go through so much?*

I didn't find meaning in this until one day when I was discussing my past with a brilliant retired physician. He told me that over the course of his career, he had been able to provide help to many patients who had previously been unable to get the help they needed from others. He credited this success with his patients not to his intellect but rather to having endured his own suffering. This suffering compelled him to learn everything he could and to care deeply about the patients he was treating.

For some people, this might have been discouraging—but for me, his revelation was enlightening. It was then that I realized I had a purpose and had been given health problems so I could overcome them and then help other people to do the same. This was my way, the way of the wounded healer. My own suffering and pain led me to solutions, and this pain reminds me of the pain and suffering my clients and readers are going through, helping me to be a better healer. Strangely, once I embraced my path as a wounded healer who was meant to overcome and help others, this helped me to accelerate my happiness and my own healing.

As you consider your current health and your Hashimoto's, can you see where it might serve a purpose in your life? Perhaps your illness is a sign from your body that you need to slow down and spend more time with your children or an aging parent. Or perhaps it's a sign that you are not living your purpose in life.

Really think about why you want to get well. Maybe your reasons are specific. Do you want to grow your hair back so that you can look great at your cousin's wedding? Do you want to have enough energy so that you can play with your kids for fifteen minutes without getting tired, or do a workout without feeling drained for days?

Don't judge yourself, and don't feel bad for your answers. It's okay and perfectly normal just to want to have nice hair or enough energy to go on a shopping spree at the mall without getting tired, or to finally fit into that sexy dress. You don't need to have grand visions of saving the world once you are well. Start with you and making yourself better, and soon enough you will find that you will want to do more good in the world.

Making Time for Yourself

Most of us are busier than ever, and that means less time to nurture ourselves. For example, a vast majority of moms don't take time for self-care. They wake up early to get their kids ready for school or nurture, feed, and chase their small children; they try to keep their significant others, parents, and in-laws happy; they say yes to the demands made on them by their boss, clients, and coworkers (no matter how difficult); and they attend children's activities and friends' parties even when they're exhausted and running on empty.

Their "free time" is spent keeping the house tidy and, if they're lucky, grooming themselves to look presentable for others, before they collapse into bed, depleted, just to do it all again the next day.

But here's the thing: no matter whether you are married or single, have kids or not, healing cannot happen if you're constantly on empty, and running on empty will eventually interfere with not just your health but also your ability to care for others. Subtle signs like feeling annoyed or overwhelmed when your spouse, children, friends, boss, or parents need something are an indication that you are not taking care of you.

Remember, an empty cup cannot fill another. You must fill your own cup first, and I encourage you to fill your cup with so much self-care that when you take the time to care for others, you will give from your overflow and you will see that giving will feel effortless. Which is why, as you're reading this book and especially when you begin the protocols, I want you to designate at least one hour to yourself each day. I know it will not be easy and that an hour sounds like an eternity, but try your best. Make this time about you and what you want to do. *But how?* you're probably asking. First, write a list of all of the things you're doing in a given day that keep you busy. Look for any time-sucking inefficiencies in your routine. Answer these questions:

- Are you going to the grocery store each day because you forgot something instead of making a four- to seven-day shopping list and meal plan?
- Are you cooking and cleaning up for two hours every day instead of batch cooking for four hours on the weekend?
- Are you getting sucked into the television set or internet for four hours instead of focusing on you?

- Are you paying your bills one by one instead of automating them?
- Are you opening up mail instead of signing up for paperless statements?
- Are you checking your email all day long instead of batch checking emails at designated times each day?
- Are you cleaning your entire house by yourself instead of hiring a housekeeper or asking family members to pitch in?
- Are you sitting in traffic on your way to and from work each day instead of taking public transportation or asking for flextime from work?

I could go on, but hopefully you get my point. Let this exercise begin to put you in the frame of mind where you consider yourself first, or at least at the top of the list. Start to think of yourself as a dear friend or family member, someone you would always make time for and drop everything to help. Are you willing to do the same for yourself?

Empathy vs. Logic

Another important step to set the stage for getting better is addressing your relationship with grief. Have you grieved your diagnosis? Have you spent too much time grieving? While it's normal to grieve after your diagnosis, research shows that spending too much time feeling sorry for yourself will block you from taking appropriate and logical action. A 2012 study from Case Western Reserve University found that empathy and logical thinking turn off one another. This means that if you're feeling sorry for yourself, you may not make the best logical decisions for your health. You may do something desperate that could potentially harm you. Or you may think that you are beyond being helped and that there is no use in trying any diet, supplement, or protocol in the world. Or you may feel powerless and look for a savior without realizing how powerful you really are.

On the other hand, empathy is also critical for anyone who is ill. Which is why, whether you were diagnosed yesterday or twenty years ago, I encourage you to take some time to grieve rather than suppressing your emotions about your condition. Show yourself the same amount of compassion that you would have for your mom, daughter, sister, or close friend—you deserve it. Take the time to comfort yourself, soothe yourself, and embrace yourself in this new journey that you are taking. And then gently get yourself ready for action.

I know it can be hard to separate your feelings from your health condition, but at times it may be helpful and even necessary. Once you've given yourself enough time to grieve, I encourage you to do your best to approach your condition as an objective scientist, implementing strategies, tracking your progress, and making modifications as needed along the way. Continue to work toward getting better, and it will happen.

Will You Be a Success Story?

In working with clients over the past few years, I've noticed several common predictors of those who eventually go on to be Hashimoto's success stories versus those who continue to struggle. Individuals who struggle often manifest the following behaviors:

- Attaching to a dogma that prevents them from getting better (*I am not going to change my diet, use medications, take supplements, or do any testing!*)
- Being unwilling to invest in themselves or necessary healing alternatives (*I will not see a doctor who doesn't take my insurance or pay for this expensive test or supplement.*)
- Doctor shopping (They get multiple opinions from multiple practitioners but don't follow through on the recommendations, or they attempt to implement multiple contradicting recommendations.)
- Perfectionism and unrealistic expectations (*I want to completely get off medications and have zero thyroid antibodies within one month of making changes after having had Hashimoto's for twenty years.*)

- Adopting "sick" as part of their identity as a way to get attention from others or to fulfill other unmet needs
- Paralysis by analysis (Someone who spends a tremendous amount of time researching their condition but doesn't take action. This person knows all about the Paleo diet, selenium, and gut infections but has yet to try the diet, buy the supplement, or get their gut tested.)
- Social isolation and lacking a support network

On the other hand, the most common behaviors in individuals who have had successful health turnarounds are as follows:

- Having a positive, can-do attitude
- Accepting the support of a loving spouse, friend, family member, or support network (*We're in this together, honey!*)
- Being grateful for small gains and improvements and celebrating little successes (*Yes! My hair stopped falling out!*)
- Dreaming big (*I have to get better; I've got books to write, mountains to climb, children to raise, and doggies to save.*)
- Doing stress-relief hobbies (yoga, writing, working out, knitting)
- Being willing to invest in themselves because they are worth it!
- Refusing to stop living just because they have Hashimoto's
- Asking for help from others
- Surrendering their need to control the situation
- Resting when they need to rest

Another essential part of the success I've seen in members of my community is having the right mind-set, which is one of a rebel, not a warrior. What's the difference? Let me explain.

Be a Rebel, Not a Warrior

I often see people using phrases like "I am suffering from [x] condition," "I am a [insert name of condition here] patient," and even "I am fighting [name of condition]." I find these phrases to be very disempowering; after all, fighting and being a warrior imply a constant struggle.

I prefer instead to think of myself and my thriving thyroid community as Root Cause Rebels. Root Cause Rebels stand up for their own health and do what's best for them, despite what society, naysayers, and the conventional medical paradigm may say.

Root Cause Rebels understand that they are unique individuals and need to make changes in their own health to get themselves better. They understand that every system is perfectly designed to achieve results and that the change has to come from them. They are leaders in making health care decisions and implementing lifestyle changes, and they don't follow the crowd. They do not compromise their knowledge, needs, or determination to heal for anyone.

Root Cause Rebels can be people who have been diagnosed with Hashimoto's, or another autoimmune condition, who want to get to the root cause of the condition. Root Cause Rebels can also be medical practitioners who know that there's much more to Hashimoto's and autoimmunity than just giving a person medications, and they understand the value of lifestyle interventions and functional medicine in restoring health.

Root Cause Rebels are willing to stand up to the status quo and say:

"I'm not going to eat like everyone else and do what everyone else is doing because I want different results than everyone else is getting."

"I want to be fit, healthy, and happy. I am not going to be pressured by commercials to eat junk food."

"I will not be told that I'm not good enough because I don't cover my face and body in chemicals."

Rebels understand the role they will play in their own recovery. When people first come to my website after being diagnosed with

Hashimoto's, the first question they often ask is, "Where can I find a doctor who can help me?" This is a smart question to ask, as having a supportive clinician who listens to you is very important, and I'm going to help you figure out how to find Dr. Right, but first I'd like to reframe this a little bit for you.

Before you find a physician to help you, start by asking: "What can I do to help myself?" After all, you know yourself best, you are the one who lives in your body and hears its subtle messages—no one else really speaks its language. You alone hold the power to change your diet, take your supplements, take your medicine, rest when you are tired, and ask for help and support when you need it. And you are the one who will take the guidance I'm offering you in this book and implement it (or not).

Finding Dr. Right

Wouldn't it be amazing if we could find the one doctor who could give us a magic pill to make all of our problems go away? We would lose weight, grow our hair back, have energy again... this might sound like a fairy tale, but it can happen and does happen for many people who get started on the correct thyroid hormones and get to the right dose. (Look at chapter 8 for more guidance on optimizing medications.)

I recommend that everyone with Hashimoto's consult with a health care professional. Even if you are extremely knowledgeable about Hashimoto's or are a health care professional yourself, it helps to have a knowledgeable, objective individual to bounce ideas off of. We all have biases and preferences that may cloud our judgment regarding our own health—thus I encourage you to find a health care professional who is open to working *with* you and willing to help you identify and resolve potential triggers of your condition. This is not the same as an unethical doctor who prescribes controlled substances to anyone who asks and who is careless with your health.

For best results, I recommend working with a functional medicine practitioner. Functional medicine clinicians approach the body as a whole; they don't focus just on the thyroid hormones. Many patients are often disappointed after going to conventional doctors who tell them that there is nothing that can be done about the autoimmune attack on the thyroid, only prescribe one type of thyroid hormone, don't dose the thyroid hormones correctly, and leave them feeling miserable!

If you're looking for a practitioner who can help you address Hashimoto's, here are some questions to ask:

1. Does the practitioner prescribe compounded thyroid medications or natural desiccated thyroid medications (NDTs like Armour Thyroid, Nature-Throid, WP Thyroid, and others)?
2. Does the practitioner prescribe low-dose naltrexone? (See page 251 for more information.)
3. Does the practitioner order adrenal saliva testing?
4. Does the practitioner have an account with functional medicine lab companies like Genova Diagnostics, Doctor's Data, ZRT Laboratory, or BioHealth Laboratory?
5. Does the practitioner order food sensitivity tests?

If you are working with a practitioner who accepts insurance, keep in mind that they may not be able to spend as much time with you as necessary due to reimbursement guidelines, and they may not be able to order functional medicine labs. While these labs can be extremely important in getting to the root cause, they are outside the standard of care and considered experimental, so most endocrinologists, primary care doctors, and internal medicine doctors will not run those tests.

Many insurance companies refuse to reimburse doctors who use "non-approved labs" or order what they deem as too many tests for a patient. Unfortunately, the insurance companies have too much control over the practice of medicine. Oftentimes, you will need to find a practitioner outside of insurance to get the care, attention, and testing you deserve. In some cases, you may be able to submit the claims to your insurance company for reimbursement. However, some insurance companies may not reimburse for these labs, so be prepared to pay out of pocket if needed.

I think of these tests as a health investment. Many of us will go out and spend money on a purse or a pair of shoes that makes us feel better in the short term, but spending money out of pocket for a lab test could dramatically improve our health in the long term.

In the event that you cannot find one doctor who will be able to prescribe medications and order the functional medicine labs, you may want to work with your medical doctor on monitoring your medications while you work with a functional medicine practitioner (who may not have prescriptive authority) to order the tests for you. If you cannot find a practitioner to order the tests for you or if you have a high deductible, you can also order the same tests on your own at a discounted price through direct-to-consumer lab companies. For a listing of direct-to-consumer lab companies, please go to www.thyroidpharmacist.com/action.

I believe that everyone needs to find a practitioner who will let them be a part of the health care team. You want someone

> who can guide you and also listen to you and your concerns. You
> want someone who is open to thinking outside the box and who
> understands that you may not fit in with the standard of care.

The Hashimoto's Protocol and How to Use This Book

My hope is that you will use this book to empower and educate yourself about Hashimoto's, including learning what the potential root
causes are and what the most important factors in healing will be. The
protocols represent the program part of this book and are designed to
be followed in the order in which they appear. The Fundamental Protocols, which include the Liver Support Protocol, the Adrenal Recovery Protocol, and the Gut Balance Protocol, will require a ninety-day
commitment from you. Here's a preview of each protocol:

LIVER SUPPORT PROTOCOL: TWO WEEKS

1. Remove potentially triggering foods.
2. Add supportive foods.
3. Reduce toxic exposure.
4. Support detox pathways.

ADRENAL RECOVERY PROTOCOL: FOUR WEEKS

1. Rest.
2. De-stress.
3. Reduce inflammation.
4. Balance the blood sugar.
5. Replenish nutrients and adaptogens.

GUT BALANCE PROTOCOL: SIX WEEKS

1. Remove reactive foods.
2. Supplement with enzymes.

3.   Balance the gut flora.
4.   Nourish the gut.

While ninety days may seem like a long time to follow a protocol, it's important to note that your condition didn't develop overnight, and it will take some time to restore your body back to health. The good news is, you will likely start feeling better within two weeks. Now that you have a good idea of how to create your own success story, let's get to it!

Welcome, my Root Cause Rebels! I am proud to be your guide and biggest cheerleader in your resistance to authority and convention. I hope the pages in this book will inspire you to take charge of your health, live well, and create your own success story.

Root Cause Reflection: Getting Ready for Action

What are your health goals?

What are your life goals?

Why do you want to be healthy?

Why do you want to achieve all of these health goals?

> *Example: I want to feel beautiful again. I want to be there for my children. I want to shine like I am meant to shine. I want to get a promotion.*

How will becoming healthy change your life for the better?

> *Example: I will wake up feeling energized, and this will help me finish the book I've dreamed about writing for years.*

What kinds of things would you do if you reached your health goals?

> *Example: I would have another baby. I would go skiing. I would train for a marathon. I would buy a sexy red dress. I would take a trip to Africa.*

What types of things do you need to do in your life to achieve these health goals?

What do you need to let go to achieve your goals?

2

Understanding the Symptoms, Diagnosis, and Origins of Hashimoto's

Before we jump into the protocol, this is the perfect moment for a deeper exploration of Hashimoto's, including the most common and confusing symptoms, the diagnosis process, and the autoimmune origins of the disease.

To start, here's a quick Thyroid 101 so you can better understand what is going on in your body and where the problem is originating. You've already learned that Hashimoto's is an autoimmune condition that affects the thyroid gland, but let's take a look at why this little butterfly-shaped organ is so important and how dysfunction of our thyroid gland can disrupt so many functions throughout the body.

The Small yet Powerful Thyroid

The thyroid gland is a small, butterfly-shaped organ that sits horizontally against the base of the neck. This important gland produces thyroid hormones, which are vital to several critical functions throughout the body. Thyroid hormones help regulate heart rate, breathing, metabolism, blood pressure, the menstrual cycle, body temperature, and much more. In fact, there's not a single cell in the body that doesn't depend on thyroid hormones in some way. In other words: trouble here can lead to trouble just about everywhere.

Through a complex chain of chemical reactions, the thyroid gland produces thyroid hormones, which are distributed throughout the body for use. Thyroid hormone disorders occur when there is too little thyroid hormone (hypothyroidism) or when there is too much thyroid hormone (hyperthyroidism). Each of these conditions can cause distinct symptoms.

Hypothyroidism = A Deficiency of Thyroid Hormone

Some of the more common symptoms of hypothyroidism produce a slowing-down effect on the body, such as sluggish metabolism leading to weight gain, fatigue, forgetfulness, cold intolerance or sensitivity to cold, depression, dry skin, constipation, loss of ambition, loss of hair, muscle cramps, stiffness, joint pain, emotional lability, loss of the outer third of the eyebrows, menstrual irregularities, infertility, and weakness.

Hyperthyroidism = An Overabundance of Thyroid Hormone

In contrast, hyperthyroidism has a stimulatory effect on the body. Classic symptoms include weight loss, palpitations, anxiety, eye protrusion, tremors, irritability, menstrual disturbances, fatigue, heat intolerance, and increased appetite. Patients may often have hair loss as well (totally not fair, I know).

If you've been newly diagnosed with Hashimoto's, you might be a bit confused by these lists of symptoms since it's very possible you have some from each. Or you might have symptoms that don't match the thyroid disorder you expected. I know I was shocked to have been diagnosed with hypothyroidism and not hyperthyroidism. In addition to feeling cold, forgetful, and tired (classical hypothyroid symptoms), I was also thin, anxious, and irritable and had heart palpitations—all of which suggested too much thyroid hormone, not too little. Because of the autoimmune nature of Hashimoto's, it operates by its own rules—which can confuse not just people with the condition, but doctors as well.

How Hashimoto's Is Unique

What I didn't realize when I was first diagnosed was that Hashimoto's has a unique set of symptoms compared to non-autoimmune hypothyroidism. In Hashimoto's, individuals can fluctuate between hypothyroid and hyperthyroid symptoms, and even experience symptoms of *both* conditions simultaneously.

In Hashimoto's, the thyroid gland is not sluggish at putting out hormones; rather, the immune system has identified thyroid cells as foreign or harmful substances and has developed antibodies to attack these cells. This attack leads to inflammation and damage of the cells that produce thyroid hormones. As the thyroid cells are damaged and destroyed by the immune system, thyroid hormones that are usually stored inside of the cells are released into circulation, leading to an excess level of thyroid hormones. This causes a transient hyperthyroidism and may even cause a toxic level of thyroid hormone in the body (known as thyrotoxicosis or Hashitoxicosis). Eventually, the extra hormone is cleared out of the body, and the person becomes hypothyroid as the damaged thyroid gland has a difficult time making enough thyroid hormone.

In this case, you might initially experience symptoms such as irritability, anxiety, and restlessness (hyperthyroidism), and then once the extra hormone gets cleared out, feelings of apathy and depression (hypothyroidism) can result. And this can happen again and again, making a person feel like they are on a roller coaster!

In addition to experiencing symptoms of hypo- and hyperthyroidism, most people with Hashimoto's also experience a variety of other inflammatory symptoms, such as irritable bowel syndrome (IBS), acid reflux, diarrhea, constipation, bloating, rashes, allergies, pain, and other nonspecific symptoms. Nutrient deficiencies, anemia, intestinal permeability, food sensitivities, gum disorders, poor stress tolerance, and hypoglycemia can occur as well. It's important to note that many of these additional symptoms or conditions are present in many other autoimmune conditions.

What's Going On in Hashimoto's

The thyroid is part of a complicated body system and does not live by itself in a vacuum. Often patients with Hashimoto's will present multiple systemic symptoms in addition to typical hypothyroid symptoms. The body becomes stuck in a chronic state of immune system overload, adrenal hormone abnormalities, gut dysbiosis, impaired digestion, impaired detoxification, inflammation, and thyroid hormone release abnormalities. This cycle is self-sustaining and will continue to cause more symptoms until an external factor intervenes and breaks the cycle apart.

Unfortunately, simply adding a synthetic thyroid medication like levothyroxine to the mix will not result in full recovery for most Hashimoto's patients and may also mask the underlying inflammation that will perpetuate the immune system imbalance and lead to other chronic conditions.

For me, it was the symptoms of gut distress that were the first clue that there might be a connection between my autoimmune condition and my intestinal health (or lack thereof). Of course, what I soon found out was that the intestines control the immune system and most diseases of autoimmunity are linked to gut health in some way. This is the reason why there is an entire Gut Balance Protocol included in the Fundamental Protocols—one of the major keys to restoring thyroid health lies in restoring the health of your intestines. Reestablishing gut health has also proven to be critical to recovery from many other autoimmune conditions.

A less obvious but equally important dysfunction in Hashimoto's is related to an impaired ability to detoxify. An impaired detoxification system is often responsible for most symptoms, preventing a person from feeling well even when other protocols are utilized. The liver is our primary detoxification organ, and this is why the Liver Support Protocol kicks off the Fundamental Protocols.

A third fundamental part of health recovery is supporting the stress response.

Root Cause Reflection:
What It Feels Like to Have Hashimoto's

I know that Hashimoto's can make you feel like you're alone and losing yourself. Many of the symptoms can feel confusing, others downright devastating. Sometimes the list of symptoms can sound more clinical than relatable, so I asked my Facebook community of Root Cause Rebels about how Hashimoto's made them feel in their own words. Here's what they said:

- "Having Hashimoto's is like living a lie; putting on your public face for a few hours here and there after you've spent the entire day feeling like you're wearing a weighted blanket, hoping no one catches you sleeping till 10:00 A.M. and napping at 2:00 P.M. and unable to remember anything on your to-do list. You're embarrassed of yourself, and it's spirit crushing."
- "I feel trapped inside. Alone in a dark cave with my dreams, but no gas/energy to carry my dreams to the world."
- "An out-of-body experience where I don't know who I am anymore, nor how I got this way. When I'm tired, I feel like there's a weight on my body preventing me from moving."
- "I feel like I'm sitting on the sidelines of life, watching everyone else enjoy their journey, wondering if I'll ever have my zest for life back."
- "Like being a clean freak but a bum is running the show."
- "To be at the mercy of an invisible illness, no control over my mood, no understandable explanation to my family on why I'm crying in the laundry room for no reason."
- "The worst part of this disease is trying to convince doctors that I am so unwell and having them tell me to eat less, exercise more, and take an antidepressant because my TSH

level is 'in the normal range.' Basically being told, 'It's all in your head. Your blood test results show you are fine. What is really going on with you is that you are unhappy in your life, nothing to do with thyroid disease.'"

- "Confusing, exasperating, numbing, exhausting. It's so incredibly hard on those who have it, as it is hard on those who love us. It's hard to explain the feelings, the desperation, the weight gain, and the lack of intimacy to those who have not experienced it firsthand. It's just hard."

While I like to focus primarily on solutions rather than the many symptoms associated with Hashimoto's, I hope that hearing about the experiences of others is validating for your own journey. Take some time to comfort yourself and show yourself kindness for what you are going through. I want you to understand that you're not going crazy, that many of your symptoms may be related to Hashimoto's, and that you can get better!

Be honest, how does Hashimoto's make you feel?

How Hashimoto's and Other Autoimmune Conditions Develop

Developing autoimmunity involves a perfect storm of events that have to line up just right. Dr. Alessio Fasano, director of the Center for Celiac Research and Treatment at Massachusetts General Hospital, found that autoimmunity develops when three factors are present:

1. Specific genes that make a person susceptible to developing autoimmune disease

2. Specific triggers that turn on the genetic expression
3. Intestinal permeability (known commonly as leaky gut) that interrupts the immune system's ability to regulate itself (This last piece may seem surprising and unrelated. However, you'll soon learn that the immune system is highly dependent on the health of the intestines.)

A person who has the genes for Hashimoto's but has not been exposed to the triggers will not develop the condition. Additionally, a person who has the genes and was exposed to the triggers but does not have intestinal permeability will not develop Hashimoto's. New research in autoimmune disease suggests that intestinal permeability always precedes autoimmunity.

Another person who has both the intestinal permeability and the triggers but not the genes will not have Hashimoto's. In this case, they may not have any symptoms at all, or they may develop a different autoimmune condition depending on their genetic background.

Bottom line is, all three *must* be present in order to develop an autoimmune condition.

Some people think that genes are destiny, but a new scientific discipline known as epigenetics shows that this is not the case. It's actually a combination of our genes and environment (which introduces triggers) that determines if we get sick or stay well. Epigenetics has shown us that we can have power over how our genes are expressed by adjusting our lifestyle choices.

Environment plays a much more profound role than genes do in Hashimoto's. For proof of this, we can look to identical twins. We know that identical twins have the same DNA, and in purely genetic conditions, there is a 100 percent concordance rate in twins. This means that if a trait or condition is 100 percent genetic, both twins would either have it or not have it. However, with respect to Hashimoto's, the concordance rate is thought to be about 50 percent. This means that if one twin has Hashimoto's, the other one only has a 50 percent chance of developing it. The twin's unique lifestyle or circumstances contribute to the development of the condition.

New research also supports the fact that autoimmunity is reversible. If one of the three factors is removed, a person will no longer present with autoimmune disease. Scientists initially demonstrated this with celiac disease, where gluten acts as both the *trigger* and the initiator of intestinal permeability. Once gluten is removed, the damaged tissue in the small intestine, which is the hallmark of celiac disease, regenerates. Then, as long as the person no longer has any additional triggers for intestinal permeability, all of the symptoms and autoimmune markers of celiac disease go away.

While Hashimoto's is a bit more complicated, with multiple triggers both inside and outside the gut, I have seen dramatic symptom improvement and remission over and over again with clients and readers who have eliminated triggers or healed their intestinal permeability. What this means for you is that even though you can't change your genes (not yet at least), you can gain control over Hashimoto's by addressing your triggers and repairing your leaky gut. I'll guide you through it.

Why Autoimmune Conditions Often Co-Occur

A person who has been diagnosed with Hashimoto's is at greater risk for other autoimmune diseases, including type 1 diabetes mellitus, celiac disease, multiple sclerosis, rheumatoid arthritis, Crohn's disease, lupus, Addison's disease, vitiligo, pernicious anemia, and many others. This is because the underlying disease mechanism is the same in each autoimmune condition, and autoimmunity can be progressive—once the immune system has begun to attack one organ, other organs may be targeted as well. Some scientists will go as far as to say that all autoimmune conditions are the same condition but with a different target. This is important to know because

Root Cause Research Corner: Origins of Autoimmunity and My Safety Theory

Scientists have developed numerous theories of how autoimmune thyroid disease may be triggered. The theories that have been proposed include the following:

Molecular mimicry theory suggests the cells of pathogens and our own thyroid look similar enough to confuse the immune system, resulting in an attack on the thyroid.

The bystander effect theorizes that an infection is present within the thyroid gland and the immune system attacks the thyroid in an attempt to kill the infecting pathogen.

Thyroid-triggered autoimmune reaction proposes that any kind of damage to the thyroid results in the gland secreting danger-associated molecular patterns or damage-associated molecular patterns (DAMPs) that recruit inflammatory cells into the thyroid and further damage the thyroid gland.

I'd also like to introduce you to the **Izabella Wentz Safety Theory** of autoimmune thyroid disease. This theory is based on the above-mentioned theories, my work and observations with Hashimoto's, and adaptive physiology.

Adaptive physiology is a concept that suggests that humans developed chronic illness to adjust to our environment and that the illness once served a protective role in the survival of our species but became maladaptive in modern times.

In cave times, our bodies adapted to intercept environmental threats as a signal that the world was a dangerous place, that it was not the best time to be adventurous or fertile, and that we needed to conserve resources.

In a way, Hashimoto's and the resultant hypothyroidism may have evolved as an adaptive mechanism to help humans conserve resources and survive in times of famine, invasion, cold weather, or disease outbreak, as the condition put them in a quasi-hibernation mode so they were more likely to retreat to their caves, survive on fewer calories, and conserve energy by sleeping more.

In modern times, nutrient depletions, inflammatory foods, stress, toxins, gut permeability, and infections can set off the same danger signal to our body and trigger the autoimmune thyroid cascade.

How can we override this signal? In simple terms, we must eliminate the things that make the immune system believe that we are in danger and that we need to conserve energy and resources.

I've found that there are universal things that everyone with Hashimoto's can do to feel better, based on my Safety Theory. This theory is the guiding principle for this book—the Fundamental Protocols and the Advanced Protocols work to send safety signals to your body by eliminating perceived threats.

in many cases, people with Hashimoto's will be told that all they need to do to get themselves well is to take thyroid hormone, yet thyroid hormone alone will not stop the progression of the autoimmune dysfunction. The good news is that the protocols in this book are designed to prevent autoimmune progression, and if you have other autoimmune conditions, you will likely see an improvement in all of them!

There are other seemingly unrelated mystery conditions that have been strongly linked to Hashimoto's, especially chronic hives and vertigo. While your doctor is likely to tell you that these conditions are unrelated and difficult to manage, I can assure you that they are very much related to Hashimoto's, and I've seen excellent results when they are treated with the Root Cause Approach.

People with Hashimoto's are more likely to develop the skin condition chronic spontaneous urticaria, also known as chronic hives, which is manifested by widespread, itchy, and swollen skin rashes. Over the last few years, I've found that people with Hashimoto's and chronic hives often have the gut protozoa *Blastocystis hominis* and that eradicating the protozoa can resolve hives, IBS, and even Hashimoto's. Scientists in Bosnia first published this connection in 2015, though I've seen it clinically since 2013.

A relationship between vestibular disorders such as vertigo and thyroid autoimmunity has been proposed. In one research study, 52 percent of Hashimoto's patients showed an alteration of vestibular function, which can affect balance and lead to vertigo and nausea. The higher the levels of thyroid peroxidase antibodies, the higher the vestibular alterations, increasing the risk of vertigo. The thyroid antibodies are thought to cross-react with parts of our vestibular system. The good news is that once you reduce the attack on your thyroid using the strategies in this book, your vertigo will improve as well.

A Definitive Diagnosis

Given the variety and number of symptoms that can be caused, either indirectly or directly, by Hashimoto's, you might think that getting a definitive diagnosis is tough—and you'd be right. Complicating matters further is the fact that many thyroid symptoms are very non-specific, which is why the medical community often disregards them in the initial stages. It's not uncommon for patients to be dismissed as having depression, stress, or anxiety and to be given antidepressants or antianxiety medications without thyroid function ever being considered. Some patients have even been misdiagnosed (and hospitalized) with bipolar disorder or schizophrenia when in fact they were suffering from thyroid imbalances.

Another common occurrence is that well-meaning doctors will test individuals for thyroid disease, but the tests will come out normal. This happens because in many cases the doctor didn't run comprehensive tests or didn't interpret the tests correctly. This is why I always have my clients ask their doctors for specific comprehensive tests and request a copy of their lab results to ensure that they are properly diagnosed. The following section will review the types of tests used to diagnose Hashimoto's.

Your Most Important Thyroid Tests

Blood tests, thyroid ultrasounds, and biopsies of the thyroid gland all can be used to diagnose Hashimoto's. Blood tests are the most easily accessible option to most people and can often uncover autoimmune thyroid disease if you do the right tests.

Most of these tests will be covered by health insurance. If your doctor will not order these tests for you, you can pay out of pocket and order them yourself through direct-to-consumer lab ordering services. For more information and a printable list of the most helpful tests and a Hashimoto's action guide, please go to www.thyroidphar macist.com/action.

TSH

The thyroid-stimulating hormone (TSH) test is used as a screening test for thyroid function. This is usually the test your doctor will run if you complain about thyroid symptoms. TSH is a pituitary hormone that sends out signals to the body to make more thyroid hormones when low levels of circulating thyroid hormone are sensed. In untreated hypothyroidism, you will eventually see abnormally elevated TSH, whereas untreated hyperthyroidism will result in an abnormally low TSH. The TSH test can serve as an excellent method for picking up long-standing thyroid abnormalities, but unfortunately it does not always catch Hashimoto's until the very late stages when a substantial amount of thyroid damage has occurred and the thyroid gland is no longer able to compensate.

In the earlier stages of Hashimoto's, a person's TSH may fluctuate between the two extremes and at times even generate normal readings. You could have a normal TSH for years while experiencing unpleasant thyroid symptoms. I often have clients come to me who have been complaining to their doctor about their symptoms such as weight gain, fatigue, and hair loss for years, and yet their thyroid-screening tests have repeatedly come back normal.

Some of the problems with this test date back to when scientists first set the normal ranges of TSH for healthy individuals. They inadvertently included elderly patients and others with compromised thyroid function in the calculations, leading to an overly lax reference range. Thus people with underactive thyroid hormones have often been told their thyroid tests are normal based on this skewed reference range.

Many labs still use the lax reference range of 0.5 to 5.0 μIU/mL where anything within that range is considered normal in the reports they provide to physicians. The majority of physicians only look for values outside the normal reference range provided by the labs and may be unfamiliar with the new guidelines. Subsequently, many doctors miss identifying patients with an elevated TSH. This is one reason why you should always ask your physician for a copy of any lab results.

The good news is that the TSH reference range is on the path toward change as a better understanding of thyroid function is gained. In recent years, the National Academy of Clinical Biochemistry indicated 95 percent of individuals without thyroid disease have TSH concentrations below 2.5 μIU/mL, and a new normal reference range was defined by the American College of Clinical Endocrinologists to be between 0.3 and 3.0 μIU/mL. Functional medicine practitioners have further defined normal reference ranges as being between 1.0 and 2.0 μIU/mL for a healthy person not taking thyroid medications.

Even with all of the redefined normal ranges, TSH screening only catches the late stage of Hashimoto's, since the body is still able to compensate in the beginning stages of thyroid dysfunction. Plus, reference ranges take into account the average values of 95 percent of the population, which means that if you are in the outlier 5 percent, you may experience symptoms of hypothyroidism or hyperthyroidism even though you have TSH values that are within the reference range. All doctors are taught the old adage "Treat the patient and not the lab tests," but sadly few conventional doctors seem to follow this advice.

I was told that my thyroid was normal when my TSH was 4.5 µIU/mL and I was exhausted, forgetful, losing hair by the handfuls, and sleeping for twelve hours each night nestled under two blankets in Southern California. I struggled with progressively worse thyroid symptoms for almost ten years before I got a diagnosis. I often wondered if I was going crazy.

I wish I had known then what was happening in my body—that I had an autoimmune disease that was continuously damaging my thyroid gland, and that the right treatment and lifestyle would not only alleviate my symptoms but also prevent further damage of my thyroid. Yet it would be almost another two years before I was diagnosed with Hashimoto's, after a different doctor tested me for thyroid antibodies, which were in the 2,000 IU/mL + range!

TPO Antibodies and TG Antibodies

The best blood tests for Hashimoto's are those that measure thyroid antibodies, which indicate an autoimmune response to the thyroid gland. The two antibody tests with elevated results in cases of Hashimoto's are:

- Thyroid peroxidase antibodies (TPO antibodies)
- Thyroglobulin antibodies (TG antibodies)

Many people with Hashimoto's will have an elevation of one or both of these antibodies. And the higher the thyroid antibodies, the greater the likelihood of developing overt hypothyroidism and possibly additional autoimmune conditions. People with Graves' disease and thyroid cancer may also have an elevation in thyroid antibodies including TPO and TG, as well as TSH receptor antibodies.

While a small number of antibodies may be present in normal individuals without thyroid disease, elevated thyroid antibodies indicate that the immune system has targeted the thyroid gland for destruction. Essentially, they are indicative of a disease process. The greater the number of antibodies, the more aggressive the attack on the thyroid gland.

Traditional doctors may not always test for Hashimoto's antibodies unless there is an elevation in TSH, which is a problem, as these antibodies can be elevated for decades before a change in TSH is seen. Doctors used to make two conclusions about a person with thyroid antibodies who did not yet have elevated TSH: they weren't likely to be experiencing any symptoms, and there was nothing that could be done for them. We now know that they were incorrect on both accounts. New research shows that the presence of thyroid antibodies can lead to symptoms like anxiety, fatigue, and a general feeling of unwellness, and lifestyle interventions have proven to reduce both symptoms and antibodies.

Current medical reports state that 80 to 90 percent of people with Hashimoto's will have TPO antibodies. That said, researchers at the University of Wisconsin Multidisciplinary Thyroid Clinic found that only half of the patients who came up positive for Hashimoto's through cytology (a test I will introduce soon) had thyroid antibodies. While current public health estimates place the incidence of Hashimoto's in the United States at somewhere in the 1 to 2 percent range, the researchers estimated that 13.4 percent of people in the United States actually have Hashimoto's and could be diagnosed with more advanced diagnostic methods.

Thyroid Ultrasound

In cases where a person does not have detectable thyroid antibodies in their blood, a thyroid ultrasound can be used to help determine a diagnosis. Clinicians have found that the changes consistent with Hashimoto's (such as tiny nodules and characteristic changes in thyroid tissue density) may be visualized on thyroid ultrasounds even when a person does not test positive for antibodies.

Yes, that means what you think—you could have Hashimoto's even if your thyroid antibody test is negative. Researchers used to believe that 90 percent of people with Hashimoto's had elevated TPO antibodies and 80 percent had elevated TG antibodies. However, new research suggests 10 to 50 percent of people with Hashimoto's may not test positive for antibodies. In this case, a person might have a less aggressive version of Hashimoto's known as antibody negative or seronegative Hashimoto's.

In many cases, thyroid ultrasounds will reveal Hashimoto's even when a person does not test positive for thyroid antibodies. However, ultrasounds are also not always definitive.

Cytology

In a cytology test, a very thin needle is inserted through the skin on the neck into the thyroid gland to remove thyroid cells. The cells are then studied under a microscope, and this examination can reveal if the cells show signs of Hashimoto's. As this diagnostic method is much more invasive than a standard blood test, it is usually reserved to determine whether thyroid nodules are benign or cancerous, not to diagnose Hashimoto's. Additionally, even this advanced test can miss Hashimoto's because only a limited number of cells are removed during cytology, and not every thyroid cell may show signs of Hashimoto's.

My friend Dr. Alan Christianson, world-renowned thyroid doctor, always says, "Tests can miss Hashimoto's. You can't completely rule out Hashimoto's unless you look at every cell inside of the thyroid gland under a microscope. This is why it's really important to listen to the patient." Thus while lab tests have their value, I also encourage each patient to work with a practitioner who can also consider the person's symptoms.

Free T3 and Free T4

The thyroid gland produces various hormones, including T1, T2, T3, T4, and calcitonin. The most active form of thyroid hormone is triiodothyronine (T3), and the next is thyroxine (T4). When they're active and circulating in the body, they're called free T3 and free T4, which can be measured by a blood test. When these levels are low but your TSH tests in the normal range, this may lead your physician to suspect a rare type of hypothyroidism known as central hypothyroidism. These hormone tests are sometimes helpful for diagnosis and often helpful when determining a correct dosage of thyroid medications. The relevance of these tests will be covered in greater depth in chapter 8.

The Five Stages of Hashimoto's

Ideally, people would be diagnosed with Hashimoto's *before* they are diagnosed with hypothyroidism—that way the risk for hypothyroidism is known and there is an opportunity to identify the underlying reasons for the immune system's attack on the thyroid. Hashimoto's progresses through five stages, which means there are several points along the way when it can be intercepted before hypothyroidism develops. For your reference, I've listed out the five stages of disease progression as well as the conventional medical approach you are likely to experience at the various stages.

- **Stage 1:** People only have the genetic predisposition to develop Hashimoto's and don't have any manifestations of the condition. They have not been exposed to the necessary autoimmune triggers, and thus their thyroid function will be optimal, with no evidence of an immune attack on the gland. They won't have any thyroid symptoms, and for all intents and purposes, they will not have any evidence of Hashimoto's outside of predisposing genes. Based on evidence I will share in chapter 4, I have come to the conclusion that up to 80 percent of people have the genetic predisposition to develop Hashimoto's if those people also encounter specific triggers. While scientists have identified *some* predisposing genes, it's important to note that the identification of disease-producing genes is still a work in progress and that genes do not determine our destiny.

- **Stage 2:** This is the beginning stage of the autoimmune attack on the thyroid. While thyroid antibody tests may be positive at this stage, all of the other thyroid blood tests will be considered within normal limits. That said, a person in stage 2 may be highly symptomatic. Doctors who don't do advanced testing often misdiagnose people in this stage with anxiety or depression, or label them as hypochondriacs.

- **Stage 3:** Here we see the beginning of thyroid gland failure; this is also known as subclinical hypothyroidism. The thyroid can no longer compensate for the autoimmune attack, so we can actually quantify changes in the traditional thyroid tests—most notably the TSH will begin to show as slightly elevated. The conventional approach at this stage is to watch and wait until the thyroid burns itself out, unless that person happens to be highly symptomatic, pregnant, or trying to conceive, or if the doctor is more progressive, synthetic thyroid hormones are prescribed. Women past their fertile period are the least likely to receive treatment at this stage, as TSH is thought to increase with age.

- **Stage 4:** At this point Hashimoto's involves overt thyroid gland failure. The thyroid can no longer make enough hormone and is not able to compensate due to advanced thyroid damage. This is the stage when most people are diagnosed by their overt symptoms and obvious out-of-range labs. Their labs are going to show an elevated TSH and low levels of T3 and T4. Most patients are likely to receive a prescription for synthetic thyroxine, such as levothyroxine (brand names include Synthroid, Levoxyl, and others).

- **Stage 5:** This stage brings progression to additional autoimmune diseases like lupus, rheumatoid arthritis, Sjogren's, psoriasis, and others.

In an ideal world, patients would be diagnosed during stage 2 so that lifestyle interventions and thyroid hormones could be started to prevent and reverse disease progression and address symptoms. Studies have found that thyroid antibodies indicative of Hashimoto's can be present for as long as a decade before the person develops impaired thyroid function. I suspect that they can be elevated for much longer, and it may take a person many decades to learn that they have hypothyroidism due to inadequate use of the TSH screening test.

Importance of Early Diagnosis

Ideally, we would want to catch thyroid antibodies before a significant amount of thyroid tissue has been damaged. This way we can look for the root cause of the autoimmune attack and slow down, reduce, and even eliminate this autoimmune attack on the thyroid.

Identifying your triggers can help to slow down and in some cases halt the autoimmune destruction of the thyroid gland. This will prevent many years of feeling unwell, having to depend on thyroid medications, and potentially developing additional autoimmune conditions.

While some people have been able to regenerate thyroid tissue and wean themselves off thyroid medications, the rates at which tissue regeneration happens are not always predictable, and of course it's much easier to prevent damage than it is to repair the gland.

Having one autoimmune condition puts us at risk for additional ones, so addressing the root cause of Hashimoto's will help prevent the development of other autoimmune conditions. In addition, several studies have shown that reducing thyroid antibody triggers can potentially prevent thyroid cancer as well.

Treatments for Hashimoto's

As discussed, the standard of care for Hashimoto's is to utilize a synthetic thyroid hormone replacement medication. Levothyroxine is the most commonly prescribed medication for Hashimoto's once a person progresses into the advanced hypothyroid stage. This is a man-made thyroid hormone that is used as replacement or supplemental therapy for internally produced thyroid hormones when our own thyroid gland cannot make enough.

While this medication can be helpful for many people and their symptoms, it does not address the underlying root causes of the condition. Synthetic thyroid meds are also often dosed incorrectly by doctors, taken incorrectly by patients, and underutilized by our bodies (due to the body's problems of converting the T4 hormone found in the pills to T3 hormone, the more physiologically active hormone). This is why many people continue to struggle with thyroid symptoms such as hair loss, brain fog, weight gain, depression, and fatigue even after they've started taking medication.

As an expert on the topic and a licensed pharmacist, I will share some best practices for getting the most from your thyroid medications. Strategies for optimizing your current medications as well as some lesser-known but often helpful methods will be discussed in chapter 8.

While people with advanced damage to their thyroid gland are usually prescribed thyroid hormone replacement, people who are in the earlier stages of Hashimoto's may be told to watch and wait and are refused thyroid hormones, despite the fact that the thyroid hormones could help them reduce symptoms and preserve thyroid function when given as early as stage 2. Instead, medications like antidepressants (for mood and fatigue) or stimulants (for brain fog, excess weight, and fatigue) are recommended. Again, these medications do not get to the underlying cause, and unlike thyroid hormones, they are often unnecessary and may have unwanted side effects.

It's important to note that the protocols outlined in this book are not intended as a substitute for thyroid medications and the standard of care, but they should be considered a complementary approach that will help you feel your best while you work with your doctor to optimize and hopefully minimize your medication. If you are experiencing many symptoms of thyroid hormone imbalance as per the assessment at the end of this chapter, you will want to refer to chapter 8 to get more guidance on working with your doctor to optimize your thyroid hormones.

Should You Consider Surgery for Hashimoto's?

A current clinical trial is under way to determine if removing the thyroid gland is associated with a better quality of life in people with Hashimoto's. While the removal of the thyroid gland results in a disappearance of thyroid antibodies, halting the attack on the thyroid, it does not guarantee that the immune system won't attack another organ. After all, the immune imbalance, which is at the root of the attack on the thyroid, will remain, even after the thyroid is removed. Additionally, removal of the thyroid requires taking lifelong medications. As many people have had so much success getting Hashimoto's into remission through lifestyle changes, I would consider removal of the thyroid gland a last resort.

Next Steps

Now that we've gone over the many symptoms of Hashimoto's, let's do an inventory of your symptoms. Completing this assessment before you start the protocols will allow us to track your progress as you begin to implement lifestyle interventions. The Fundamental Protocols will help most of these symptoms. Fatigue, mood, and stomach issues may be the first symptoms to resolve, while hair regrowth and weight loss may be a more gradual process.

Thyroid Symptom Assessment

Which of the following thyroid symptoms do you have?

Rate your symptoms on a scale of 1 to 10, where 1 means you do not experience the symptom at all, 10 means it drastically affects your lifestyle, and n/a means it doesn't apply to you. I recommend that you come back to this assessment after completing each protocol to track improvements.

Fatigue/Drowsiness	1 2 3 4 5 6 7 8 9 10 n/a
Hair Loss	1 2 3 4 5 6 7 8 9 10 n/a
Cold Intolerance	1 2 3 4 5 6 7 8 9 10 n/a
Inability to Lose Weight	1 2 3 4 5 6 7 8 9 10 n/a
Sadness/Depression	1 2 3 4 5 6 7 8 9 10 n/a
Mental Fog/Forgetfulness	1 2 3 4 5 6 7 8 9 10 n/a
Joint Pain	1 2 3 4 5 6 7 8 9 10 n/a
Acne	1 2 3 4 5 6 7 8 9 10 n/a
Puffy Face	1 2 3 4 5 6 7 8 9 10 n/a
Acid Reflux	1 2 3 4 5 6 7 8 9 10 n/a
Stomach Pain	1 2 3 4 5 6 7 8 9 10 n/a
Morning Fatigue	1 2 3 4 5 6 7 8 9 10 n/a
Irritability	1 2 3 4 5 6 7 8 9 10 n/a
Palpitations	1 2 3 4 5 6 7 8 9 10 n/a
Night Sweats	1 2 3 4 5 6 7 8 9 10 n/a
Emotional Lability	1 2 3 4 5 6 7 8 9 10 n/a
Weight Loss	1 2 3 4 5 6 7 8 9 10 n/a
Nervousness	1 2 3 4 5 6 7 8 9 10 n/a
Anxiety	1 2 3 4 5 6 7 8 9 10 n/a
Feeling Hot	1 2 3 4 5 6 7 8 9 10 n/a
Trouble Sleeping	1 2 3 4 5 6 7 8 9 10 n/a
Apathy/Feeling Numb	1 2 3 4 5 6 7 8 9 10 n/a
Vertigo	1 2 3 4 5 6 7 8 9 10 n/a
Nausea	1 2 3 4 5 6 7 8 9 10 n/a

What additional symptoms do you experience?

A Plan for Healing

Now that you've done an inventory of your symptoms, it's time to create a plan for healing. Chapter 3 will outline how the Root Cause Approach can help you not just eliminate your symptoms but also reverse your condition by addressing the root cause.

3

How the Root Cause Approach Can Help You Recover Your Health

While understanding the origins of your Hashimoto's can be complicated, getting your health back doesn't have to be. One of the most important lessons I've learned over the years is that while each person's Hashimoto's is different, there are strategies that have been proven successful across the board. The approach you'll discover in *Hashimoto's Protocol* incorporates these proven strategies, providing you with a clear and simple path to reducing and eliminating many common symptoms.

Over the last several years, I've focused my work exclusively on the Hashimoto's population, and this narrow focus has allowed me to streamline the Root Cause Approach since it was introduced in my first book. The more I have learned about Hashimoto's, the more I've realized that symptoms can be greatly improved by addressing underlying issues in a specific order, starting with general vulnerabilities like impairments in the liver's detox capabilities, stress hormone imbalances, and digestive challenges, and then moving into individual triggers such as infections and toxins.

First, we must address what I refer to as your Achilles' heel vulnerabilities, or weaknesses within the body. These vulnerabilities can develop when the body is not properly fed, is overstressed, or is exposed to toxins. These situations lead to nutrient depletions, food sensitivities, inflammation, an impaired stress response, an inability to handle toxins, intestinal permeability, and result in the body losing its ability to regulate and repair itself. This is why the main focus of my Fundamental Protocols is to add supportive strengthening nourishment while removing common, everyday stressors and sources of inflammation to make the body stronger and more resilient. Most people feel significantly better within a short period of adding nourishment and removing environmental stressors.

Once we've addressed the vulnerabilities, we move into the Advanced Protocols, which focus on identifying and removing significant and often unique triggers, optimizing thyroid hormone levels, and further adjusting nutrition and the stress response if needed.

While it's important for you to be aware of the potential triggers that may have led to the development of Hashimoto's, I'm going to save this investigation for later in the book. My experience in working with patients with Hashimoto's has proven that a focus on the many triggers can put a person into a state of paralysis by analysis, and trying to understand and explore all of the potential triggers can sometimes delay healing rather than accelerate it. It can become too tempting to focus completely on the digging rather than the doing, and the doing is what is going to start making you feel better faster. Thus rather than focusing on the possible problems, I want you to start implementing the many solutions that we know work.

I will guide you through a deeper exploration of triggers when we reach the Advanced Protocols, where you will take a series of assessments that will tell you if you need to work through the later, more specific protocols.

While the prospect of unique triggers may seem daunting, I've found that unique triggers can generally be classified into three main categories: stress, infections, and toxins.

Not everyone with Hashimoto's will have underlying infections that need to be removed before recovery or remission can happen. But if you do, getting to the bottom of an infection can demand a bit of

Root Cause Reflection: What Was Going On in Your Life Before You Got Sick?

Whenever I'm working with a new client, we go through an intake process of uncovering potential triggers and exacerbating factors that have led them to a path of disease. The goal of this exercise is to identify the wrong turns so we can start making some right turns toward a path to wellness.

When I conducted a survey of my readers with Hashimoto's in 2015, I focused one of the questions on what had been happening before readers started to feel unwell. With this information, I wanted to see if we could uncover the most common predisposing triggers. Out of the two-thousand-plus responses, stress seemed to be the most common answer, but there were other elements and experiences that preceded and possibly contributed to a Hashimoto's diagnosis as well. I am sharing this list with you to help you uncover your own predisposing triggers. Readers reported the following events in their lives just before they started to feel unwell:

69% a lot of stress

23% having a baby

20% moving to a new home

17% suffering the death of a loved one

11% mononucleosis, caused by the Epstein-Barr virus

11% exposure to a toxin

8% extensive dental work

6% a car accident

5% remodeling their home

4% food poisoning (potential gut infection)

4% possible exposure to the bacteria that causes Lyme disease through a tick bite

2% breast augmentation surgery

You can see that there are a variety of predisposing factors that can ignite the autoimmune response in those who are genetically predisposed to it. While all of these triggers may seem diverse, when we take a step back, we can see that they all involve stress, toxins, or infections. From a holistic perspective, these are the three main pathways to illness.

What was going on in your life when you got sick?

For a downloadable workbook of the Root Cause Reflection excerpts, please go to www.thyroidpharmacist.com/action.

detective work and often requires consulting with a health care professional, ordering extensive laboratory tests, and taking expensive medications or supplements. (Unfortunately, some or all of these endeavors may not be covered by insurance due to their "experimental" nature.)

Everyone has toxins in their body, to some degree. Our modern world is full of them, so they are essentially unavoidable. The difference between acceptable toxins and harmful toxins lies in a few different factors. One of the most critical factors is the existing level of toxicity in the body. The higher our toxic load, the more likely toxins will interfere with our immune and endocrine functions. The other factor is whether we are individually sensitive to the toxin. In the case when someone is genetically or otherwise predisposed to be ultrasensitive to a toxin, even small amounts in the person's body or environment will cause the person to fall ill.

I intentionally have you focus on vulnerabilities before addressing infections and toxins because sometimes fixing vulnerabilities can help you overcome your unique triggers without requiring any additional intervention. Furthermore, skipping the fundamentals and going straight for the triggers may result in toxin recirculation and reinfection. The Fundamental Protocols will focus first on patching up any vulnerabilities you may have and then you can do the finishing work by addressing triggers. Everyone with Hashimoto's, regardless of their root cause, can benefit from the ground-level improvements that will be established by completing the three Fundamental Protocols.

The Fundamental Protocols

The first part of the Root Cause Approach, the Fundamental Protocols, focuses on strengthening your body so it can properly repair itself. We will achieve this by: nourishing your body with real food; removing reactive foods; adding minerals and vitamins that your body may be missing; putting your body in a relaxed, healing state; and supporting your body's natural processes and defenses.

These interventions are lifestyle changes. While you may spend some more money on buying quality foods and supplements, these interventions are relatively inexpensive to implement but will take effort and commitment on your part. The great news is that most people feel much better almost immediately after starting these lifestyle changes, and some people, just by supporting their body's own healing capabilities, will be able to get Hashimoto's into remission.

Your body will be strengthened by following these three protocols:

- **Liver Support Protocol:** This two-week kickoff will guide you on how to eliminate hidden toxins from your everyday life and how to help your liver process out the toxins you may have in your body. Both are critical steps for anyone who's had problems with taking supplements or is struggling with current symptoms. Most people see drastic changes just by completing this step alone.
- **Adrenal Recovery Protocol:** Here, you will learn how to support your stress hormones and embrace mind-set and stress-reduction techniques that will help shift your body into a

regenerative process so you can become stronger and more resilient.

- **Gut Balance Protocol:** In this final Fundamental Protocol, I will teach you how to optimize your gut health and renew bacterial and microbial balance in the gut so you can start healing from within.

You might wonder why we start with the liver when the gut is always an issue for people with Hashimoto's. While I didn't start with liver support myself, nor did I start clients there in my early work with Hashimoto's protocols, I've found over time that it is absolutely the most effective place to start.

I used to look for the most obvious root causes and imbalances and address those first, but sometimes improvements took a long time to see. Once I started my clients with liver support, I found that this allowed most of my clients to feel better within just a few short weeks, even those who had been working with other practitioners for months and years. I saw more profound improvements in multiple chemical sensitivities, hormonal imbalances, rashes, joint pains, mood swings, fatigue, and brain fog within two weeks of utilizing the Liver Support Protocol than I had ever seen when my clients were primarily focused on trigger identification for months at a time.

Now, anyone who comes to me with Hashimoto's will be started on liver support first before they move on to any other protocol. The Liver Support Protocol has become my secret sauce and has helped the majority of my clients feel significantly better in as little as a week.

The Advanced Protocols

The second set of protocols focuses on identifying and addressing your unique triggers. Contrary to reports you may have seen online of people who have said that gluten was their only root cause, most people will have multiple root causes. Hashimoto's is often a combination of

Fundamental Healing

In a nutshell, we will focus on utilizing food as medicine (or food pharmacology, as I like to call it), coupled with targeted supplements and lifestyle changes that restore health during the Fundamental Protocols.

The Fundamental Protocols will introduce you to targeted interventions that will be modified along the way, adjusting your supplements and nutrition within each of the three phases of the protocol. You'll be introduced to three diets (Root Cause Intro, Paleo, and Autoimmune Diets) to go with the protocols. While each of the protocols is distinct, they do have the following core concepts in common:

- They limit reactive and processed foods like gluten, dairy, soy, caffeine, and sugar.
- They're rich in vegetables—meals should be 25 percent meat and 75 percent vegetables, and you should aim for six cups of veggies and fruit each day.
- They stress the inclusion of foods low on the glycemic index to help balance blood sugar and adrenal issues, which are often implicated in Hashimoto's. This includes limiting fruit to fewer than two servings per day.
- They recommend that you eat a variety of foods and rotate them. If you have a leaky gut, eating the same foods over and over, no matter how healthy, will lead to the sensitivity to those foods. Rotating foods is an excellent way to prevent new food reactions and to improve nutrient sufficiency.
- They emphasize the importance of nutrient density. Aim to get most of your foods from organic meat and veggies, green smoothies, green juices, bone broth, liver, fermented foods, and gelatins.

> • They suggest limiting seaweed due to its immune-modu-
> lating abilities and high iodine content.
> • They remind you to eat foods rich in good fats to support
> hair, skin, and blood sugar.

food sensitivities, an impaired ability to handle stress, difficulty han-
dling toxins, a leaky gut, a lack of thyroid hormone, infections, and
nutrient depletions. A secret some people may not know is that your
body needs to be strengthened in order to address triggers properly
and effectively.

Here's a glimpse at what we'll cover in the Advanced Protocols
(important reminder: these protocols are to be done on an as-needed
basis—not everyone will need to complete every single protocol to
feel better):

- **Protocols for Optimizing Thyroid Hormones:** I'll walk you
  through the most important lab testing as well as how to understand your lab results. Furthermore, this protocol addresses the
  use of medications, including common concerns related to which
  ones, how and when to take them, at what dose, and how to
  convert between medications. We also cover tissue-regenerating
  protocols that can help heal your thyroid gland. If you are not
  yet taking thyroid hormones and had a high score on the Thyroid Symptom Assessment, consider making the interventions
  in this chapter a priority.
- **Protocols for Mastering Nutrition and Nutrients:** We will
  take a deeper dive into nutrition and nutrients, identify any
  remaining sensitivities or deficiencies you may have, and address
  how to supplement appropriately.
- **Protocols for Overcoming Traumatic Stress:** We'll explore

advanced reasons for stress dysfunction, how to test for it, and how to finally heal it!

- **Protocols for Addressing Infections:** We'll dig deep into chronic infections—which often trigger Hashimoto's through molecular mimicry—how to test for them, and how to treat them. I share natural, herbal, dietary, and pharmaceutical options that have worked with my clients.
- **Protocols for Removing Toxins:** I'll help you identify toxins in food and environment that may still be affecting you. We'll also look for any dental triggers you may have and how to address them. These are frequently overlooked but so important!

The Root Cause Guidelines for Success

Just as I recommend that you keep a written progress of your interventions and improvements in a journal, I've kept a record of progress notes on my clients over the years to record what's been the most effective—and you'll be following the results of this record when you begin the protocols in the next chapter.

There are, however, other guidelines for success I've encountered that I'd like to share with you before you begin. These are mind-set suggestions and general guidance that I think you'll find helpful.

Use what you can use and leave the rest. I've written this book as a reference and also as a healing protocol that can help the greatest number of people with Hashimoto's. That means for some of you, there will be more here than you need, and for others, there won't be enough. Most people won't need to implement every single recommendation in this book, though I do recommend that all of you follow the Fundamental Protocols.

I've purposely left some of the research and studies out of this book. I could have easily written a thousand-page book on Hashimoto's, but I wanted this book to be more approachable. My previous book, *Hashimoto's Thyroiditis: Lifestyle Interventions for Finding and Treating the Root Cause,* dives deep into the research and theory and offers a more comprehensive look. There was just too much to cover in this book to include all that *and* make it user friendly!

Let me be your bridge. You might have noticed that I'm a pharmacist whose approach to healing doesn't rely on pharmaceutical medications. The main reason for this is that conventional medicine didn't have an answer for reversing my Hashimoto's, so the solution I developed was built instead around practices found in natural medicine. That doesn't mean medications don't have their appropriate time, place, and use. In fact, conventional, natural, integrative, and functional medicine methods can all fill an important role in creating health. What's important is that you have an open mind about what might work for you.

I didn't used to have an open mind. I was wary of the use of any diets, supplements, and testing that were not FDA approved; I thought that the FDA knew everything. But years of working in public health, self-experimentation, and watching people actually getting better with "unapproved" methods have completely changed my mind.

By the same token, I've also seen some dangerous practices within the natural medicine world. I've witnessed practitioners telling people to forgo medications in potentially life-threatening situations or suggesting that if a person just decided that they didn't have a condition, they would be healed. I have also seen claims of cure-all diets, supplements, and plans, which are irresponsible and potentially dangerous practices.

I don't subscribe to dogmas. I believe that dogmas are dangerous. In fact, I often tell my clients not to be a martyr to a sole healing philosophy. In my experience, an integrative and patient-centered approach to healing is usually the most effective approach (and also the kindest, as it doesn't prolong unnecessary suffering). This means always question a practitioner who claims that there's only one way to feeling better with a condition, whether it's "just medications," "just diet," or "just supplements." The truth is that there is not just one way of helping every single person feel better and recover their health. Everyone is different and may require different interventions throughout their journey.

By popular demand, I have listed specific dietary protocols, recipes, supplements, tests, and medications that I have found to be most helpful in treating my clients. This does not mean that other protocols developed by other practitioners won't work, but I recommend only accepting guidance from a practitioner you trust, a person who has a track record of success with other Hashimoto's patients.

In my work, including what you'll find here in this book, I have done my best to be a bridge between the conventional and natural medical world, taking the best from both worlds to give you the safest and most effective ways you can help yourself feel better. Let me be your bridge to recovery!

The motivation has to come from you. While this book, a doctor, or a health coach can tell you exactly what you need to do to get better, the motivation to get better has to come from you. I modeled this book after my client work and my twelve-week Hashimoto's self-management program that has seen great success with many of my clients. Each of my Root Cause Rebels walks away from the program with the necessary information to get Hashimoto's in remission. However, the ones who truly become success stories are the ones who are motivated to implement the changes we discuss here.

Patience and persistence are required. The change in your health won't happen because of any one book, course, or consultation. It will come about only through your continuous efforts to keep digging. It starts with you and your commitment to your health. As you follow the protocols I've outlined in this book, you will not only create a better you, but you also help create a better life for those around you.

It's important to note that most people with Hashimoto's have multiple root causes, not just one. This means that there is often quite a bit of trial and error and peeling back the layers of the onion to get to the core of the problem. The protocols will help guide you through that peeling process, but you will need to be the one who provides the persistence and patience, both of which will be essential as your unique system reveals its Hashimoto's story.

Remember that you know yourself best and only you can be the empowered patient. It's up to you to track your symptoms, interventions, and side effects, and to speak up if you notice any changes in your health that need medical attention. This is especially true when it comes to any medications you may be taking. Remember that you know yourself best, and please use common sense. If you think something your doctor is recommending is not working, speak up! If the protocols in this book are making you feel worse instead of better, listen to your body and discontinue what doesn't serve you.

Start with the Fundamental Protocols and add the Advanced Protocols when you're ready. The Fundamental Protocols have been designed to provide you with a solid groundwork for healing and can in many cases result in a complete remission of symptoms and the condition. If you think you may be an advanced case, you can start exploring the Advanced Protocols as you work through the Fundamental Protocols. However, for best results, please note that the Fundamental Protocols are a prerequisite to the Advanced Protocols for removing toxins.

Achieving the Dream of Health

I once heard the saying "A person who has their health has a hundred dreams. A person who doesn't, has just one." I don't know what specific symptoms you're dealing with or how long you've been suffering, but I know that having Hashimoto's can feel like you are trapped alone in a dark cave with your dreams but with no way out and no energy to carry your dreams to the world. I want to let you know that there is a light at the end of the tunnel. You don't have to suffer and feel like you are losing out on life. While I've shared some statistics of improvements, I'd like to share a couple of stories of clients who have recovered their health and have been able to follow their dreams!

Getting Support: Your Healing Team

I am a big believer that every person with Hashimoto's needs to be their own health advocate, but it's so much easier to be your own advocate when you've got support! Here's who you should have on your healing team:

- **You:** The educated and empowered patient, you are the most important part of your healing team.
- **Physician:** An open-minded and supportive physician who can monitor your condition and prescribe medications will be crucial.
- **Functional medicine practitioner:** This could be a medical doctor, a chiropractor, a naturopathic physician, an acupuncturist, a nutritionist, a nurse practitioner, or a consultant pharmacist. The functional medicine practitioner will address your health through a whole-body approach.
- **Compounding pharmacist:** This specialized pharmacist will offer a wealth of knowledge and be your best bet for getting medications tailored to your individual needs.
- **Biological dentist:** More than a standard dentist, a biological dentist understands that the health of your mouth can affect the health of your entire body.
- **Health coach:** This professional can guide you, support you, and motivate you in your health journey.
- **Support network:** Your community will be beneficial to you whether you're new to Hashimoto's or you've been dealing with it for a while. Your support network can be in the form of family members, friends, a coach, a therapist, or a group.
- **Me!:** I hope this book, my Facebook page, and the *Thyroid Pharmacist* blog will serve as another place for you to find

> support. I've also developed a number of additional re-
> sources specifically for people with Hashimoto's that I will
> mention later in this book.

One of them is about my client Susan, who, at forty-six, had spent ten years suffering from multiple chemical sensitivities and three years working on overcoming Hashimoto's. After completing my two-week liver support, she was able to reduce her multiple chemical sensitivities by half! For the first time in almost five years, she was able to go Christmas shopping at the mall with her teenage girls. She was excited to finally be able to walk past a Yankee Candle store without feeling sick.

Another is about a woman named Leslie. Leslie was thirty-three when she joined my beta Hashimoto's self-management program. Participants in this program filled out intake forms and progress reports, and had consults with me to make sure they were seeing improvements in their health. Leslie's initial intake form indicated a long laundry list of symptoms including polycystic ovary syndrome (PCOS), sleep apnea, depression, eczema, irritable bowel syndrome (IBS), hair loss, and sleeping for fifteen hours each night.

When it came time for our consult, Leslie kept postponing, and I became concerned that maybe she was struggling with the program or her symptoms. It turned out that she was still working through the program on her own and was very much making progress! When we finally had our consult six months later, I was elated to hear that her troubles with IBS, PCOS, eczema, sleep apnea, and hair loss were gone! Her depression had improved (she was also getting help from a therapist), and she was feeling energetic after nine hours of sleep instead of fifteen. Her thyroid antibodies were in the remission range, and her hair had started growing back. I went back to the list of symptoms and saw that everything listed was now resolved or was on its way there.

"Well, what else can I help you with?" I asked.

She replied, "I never thought I'd be able to become a mom with all of my health issues, but now I think this dream is possible. Can you recommend a good prenatal vitamin and give me some guidelines on optimal thyroid medication dosing during pregnancy?" My heart was overflowing with joy that she was not just feeling better but also was now able to make one of her lifelong dreams a reality!

Hundreds of others have shared information with me about their success with my programs. Graduates of my twelve-week course (which is the basis for this book) who took a survey afterward shared their results, summarized here:

97% improved their knowledge of Hashimoto's

81% saw an improvement or resolution in depression

80% saw a reduction in stomach pain

75% saw a reduction in joint pain

74% saw an improvement in fatigue

73% saw a reduction in TSH

71% improved their acid reflux

65% saw an improvement in symptoms after the liver cleanse

62.5% reported reduced brain fog

61% reduced their irritability

58% reduced their forgetfulness

56% reduced their TPO antibodies

54% reduced their palpitations

53% improved weight loss

52% saw an improvement in morning energy

50% reduced night sweats

45% reduced hair loss

45% saw improvement in insomnia

44% saw a reduction in TG antibodies

42% saw an improvement in nervousness and anxiety

Susan's and Leslie's stories and these survey results represent only a small sampling of some of the success stories from people who have been able to overcome Hashimoto's using the programs I've designed. Many of my clients have been complicated cases with a multitude of symptoms, and many have recovered and followed their dreams. It's been an honor to be a guide in their journey back to health (and back to feeling like themselves again!). As you get ready to start the protocols, I hope you'll step forward with great hope, optimism, and enthusiasm about the journey ahead of you.

PART II

THE FUNDAMENTAL PROTOCOLS

Welcome to the Fundamental Protocols. If you were eager to get started and jumped right to this section, you missed a lot about what each protocol addresses, how they were developed, and why they're in the order that they are. And that's okay; I don't blame you for wanting to get right to the feeling-better process! I do, however, want you to have a basic understanding of what's to come because it will give you confidence in the path that has been laid out before you.

As a reminder, the Fundamental Protocols include the Liver Support Protocol, the Adrenal Recovery Protocol, and the Gut Balance

Protocol. You will complete these three protocols over ninety days, during which time you will strengthen your body and restore its ability to heal itself. We will accomplish this by using food as medicine, incorporating strategic supplements, and making lifestyle changes that will help put your body in a relaxed, healing state.

The protocols will focus on the liver, the adrenal glands, and the gut. My research and experience—both personal and with clients—has revealed these three areas represent a sort of axis of thyroid-related autoimmunity.

We will direct our attention first to the liver, as many symptoms of Hashimoto's can be linked to an impaired detoxification system (and the liver is our primary detoxification organ). Next, I will guide you through a protocol designed to help you recover optimal adrenal function. Most people with autoimmune thyroid disease have altered adrenal hormone activity, which can both worsen thyroid symptoms and act as a trigger of thyroid disease. Steps taken in this second protocol will help reset your internal stress response. Finally, we will focus on reestablishing balance in the gut. A common condition seen in autoimmunity is intestinal permeability (aka leaky gut), which interrupts the immune system's ability to regulate itself. This dysregulation can put the body into a perpetual attack mode that will be counterproductive to your healing.

You will find that each protocol is packed with detailed guidance and information, in some cases, more than you might want! My advice is to use only what you need now and save the rest for later. Keep in mind that every step and strategy in this section has been vetted and tested by me and wouldn't be here unless it were absolutely necessary to your recovery. Now, let's get to healing.

4

Liver Support Protocol

Our modern world exposes us to an unprecedented number of toxins every day. We inhale toxins through the air we breathe, absorb them through our skin when we use personal care products, and ingest them when we eat foods that have been steeped in pesticides. New, unregulated chemicals are constantly introduced into our society without any consideration for long-term effects on us or our planet.

People with Hashimoto's often have an impaired ability to handle all these toxins. This may occur for a variety of reasons. You could have a genetic predisposition to be less efficient at detoxification, nutrient deficiencies, an overburdened system, or excessive exposure to toxins, any of which can compromise the body's natural detox pathways.

While numerous heavy-duty toxins have been implicated in potentially triggering Hashimoto's and causing endocrine imbalances, some people may never be exposed to heavy toxins but may have the perfect storm of vulnerabilities that will lead to a greater accumulation of toxins. In general, people who develop autoimmune diseases are more sensitive to toxins in the environment—we are the canaries in the coal mines, and our symptoms are the signs of the invisible dangers that surround us.

How do you know if you have an impaired ability to process toxins? We have to determine whether you're exhibiting symptoms of impaired liver function. The liver is our main detoxification organ and can become congested from the countless toxic substances we are exposed to on a daily basis. A congested liver is one of the many reasons why people's bodies don't utilize their thyroid medications effectively and don't convert T4 to the active T3 hormone correctly. A congested liver can also lead to a greater buildup of toxins, an issue that might create new symptoms altogether or worsen those you might already be experiencing as a result of Hashimoto's. My experience has taught me that supporting the liver is an important part of reestablishing healthy thyroid function and eliminating the many symptoms associated with Hashimoto's.

Liver dysfunction can present itself in many different types of signs and symptoms, including digestive problems, extreme sensitivity to supplements or medications, fatigue, skin breakouts, and more. I've designed the liver assessment to reflect a more comprehensive list of all the potential symptoms. Completing this assessment will help establish your current level of toxicity. You will also repeat this assessment after you have completed the two-week liver protocol.

LIVER ASSESSMENT

Mark which symptoms apply to you.

- ☐ Acne
- ☐ Anger, irritability, or aggressiveness
- ☐ Anxiety, fear, or nervousness
- ☐ Apathy, lethargy
- ☐ Arthritis
- ☐ Asthma, bronchitis
- ☐ Bags or dark circles under eyes
- ☐ Bad breath
- ☐ Belching or passing gas
- ☐ Binge eating or drinking
- ☐ Bloating
- ☐ Blurred or tunnel vision
- ☐ Brain fog
- ☐ Canker sores
- ☐ Chest congestion
- ☐ Chest pain
- ☐ Chronic coughing
- ☐ Compulsive eating
- ☐ Confusion, poor comprehension
- ☐ Constipation
- ☐ Craving certain foods
- ☐ Depression
- ☐ Diarrhea
- ☐ Difficulty breathing
- ☐ Difficulty in making decisions
- ☐ Digestive problems

☐ Dizziness
☐ Drainage from ear
☐ Earaches, ear infections
☐ Eczema
☐ Emotional dysregulation
☐ Excessive mucus formation
☐ Excessive sweating
☐ Excessive weight
☐ Faintness
☐ Fatigue, sluggishness
☐ Feeling of weakness or tiredness
☐ Food sensitivities
☐ Flushing or hot flashes
☐ Frequent illness
☐ Frequent or urgent urination
☐ Gagging, frequent need to clear throat
☐ Genital itch or discharge
☐ Hair loss
☐ Hay fever
☐ Headaches
☐ Heartburn
☐ Hives, rashes, or dry skin
☐ Hormonal imbalances
☐ Hyperactivity
☐ Insomnia
☐ Intestinal or stomach pain
☐ Irregular or skipped heartbeat
☐ Itchy ears
☐ Learning disabilities
☐ Mood swings
☐ Multiple chemical sensitivity

☐ Nausea or vomiting
☐ Near- or farsightedness
☐ One or more autoimmune conditions
☐ Pain or aches in joints
☐ Pain or aches in muscles
☐ Poor concentration
☐ Poor memory
☐ Poor physical coordination
☐ Rapid or pounding heartbeat
☐ Restlessness
☐ Ringing in ears, hearing loss
☐ Sensitivity to medications and supplements
☐ Shortness of breath
☐ Sinus problems
☐ Slurred speech
☐ Sneezing attacks
☐ Sore throat, hoarseness, loss of voice
☐ Stiffness or limitation of movement
☐ Stuffy nose
☐ Stuttering or stammering
☐ Swollen, reddened, or sticky eyelids
☐ Swollen or discolored tongue, gum, lips
☐ Underweight
☐ Unexplained weakness
☐ Water retention
☐ Watery or itchy eyes

Total number of symptoms: ____

<3:   Optimal
3–12:   Mild toxicity
13–24: Moderate toxicity
>25:   Severe toxicity

If you scored high on this scale, don't worry, you're not alone. Many people with Hashimoto's are likely to end up with a high toxicity score in the beginning stages of their journeys before they start to make changes.

Whenever I see a high toxicity score in my clients, I see this as a big opportunity for improvement, knowing that once you remove some of the toxins from your life, you'll start to feel better. How do I know this? Because after utilizing the Liver Support Protocol with hundreds of people with Hashimoto's, I've found that 65 percent of them feel significantly better after implementing it.

The Liver Support Protocol will help you even if the assessment suggested that you had only mild toxicity. This is because it's designed to reduce your toxic burden and teach you how to support your body's own detox pathways. These are steps that will make you more resilient to the chemical warfare your body faces in our environment.

Supporting the liver first is especially important in autoimmunity, and in Hashimoto's in particular. Since a permeable gut can lead to impaired detox abilities and hypothyroidism can result in a decreased ability to sweat, people with Hashimoto's are more prone to developing a chemical backlog in the body. After working with numerous clients, I've discovered that people who do not begin with liver support (and instead start with the gut or adrenals) are more likely to react to medications, supplements, and even foods. Supporting the liver can really kick-start your healing, and it also makes you feel brighter, happier, and more alive.

So let's take a look at the ways we can support your liver.

What Is the Liver Support Protocol?

My liver support program is a two-week protocol that focuses on reducing your exposure to toxic substances while simultaneously supporting the liver to allow for a faster clearance of toxins out of the body. The Liver Support Protocol is gentle and effective because it is based on natural principles, utilizing real food as part of the Root

Cause Intro Diet, nutrients, and gentle herbs to strengthen your body while also guiding you on how to reduce your daily toxic exposures. The gentle Liver Support Protocol has four steps:

1. Remove potentially triggering foods.
2. Add supportive foods.
3. Reduce toxic exposure.
4. Support detox pathways.

I want to emphasize the word *gentle* here (you might have noticed I used it a few times!) because it distinguishes some of what's different about my Liver Support Protocol compared to others out there. This protocol is not the same as a forceful detox, juice fast, or chelation protocol. My liver support does not utilize coffee enemas, high doses of iodine, fasting, or putting your body in dangerous situations. While these types of interventions may be a helpful way for some people to address their health needs, they can make many people with autoimmune thyroid disease feel worse (especially when done without medical supervision). This is because they can pull toxins out from storage within the body at an aggressive rate, which can overwhelm the detox pathways that are already overburdened due to Hashimoto's.

Forceful detox methods may lead to potentially serious consequences:

- Blood sugar dysregulation, fainting, or weakness with juice fasting or the elemental diet used for small intestinal bacterial overgrowth (SIBO)
- Rashes, weakness, and new autoimmune reactions with chelation protocols, even when using natural chelating agents like spirulina and chlorella
- Bowel perforation, colitis (colon inflammation that may lead to hospitalization), and pain with coffee enemas

- Increased thyroid gland destruction, depletion of thyroid hormones, a dramatic increase of thyroid antibodies leading to debilitating fatigue, brain fog, palpitations, anxiety, and hair loss with high doses of iodine, which cause a rapid release of toxins from the thyroid gland

While some old-school natural practitioners have found the above methods helpful, my research and experience have led me to believe that in the modern world, these interventions may be more harmful than they have been in the past. I believe that this is due to the following factors:

- **Higher toxic load:** People with autoimmune disease today seem to have a higher toxic load combined with a reduced ability to handle the toxins. A forceful detox method can overwhelm our detoxification system with more toxins than the system can clear, resulting in toxins circulating in the bloodstream (which causes inflammation) and depositing in other parts of the body (which may result in an autoimmune response in a new organ like the brain, pancreas, or liver).
- **Altered adrenal hormone activity:** Most people with autoimmune thyroid disease have altered adrenal hormone activity. Adrenal hormones are also known as stress hormones and tame our inflammation. Mobilized toxins produce inflammation, and if left unchecked, this inflammation can lead to an exacerbation of symptoms such as fatigue, pain, and headaches.
- **Intestinal permeability:** Every autoimmune condition is associated with intestinal permeability. This impaired gut function leads to a reduced absorption of nutrients required for detoxification as well as a reduced excretion of toxins. This is especially true with constipation, which holds toxins in the body, but also with diarrhea, where the toxins are more likely to end up in the bloodstream due to intestinal permeability.

Detoxing Too Early Can Be Harmful

Back when I was in the thick of things, I tried detoxing with spirulina, and I developed a new autoimmune condition called giant papillary conjunctivitis. I developed giant pimples on the inside of my eyelids, and it was awful! After that point I was no longer able to wear my contact lenses and had to resort to wearing either glasses or the expensive daily disposable contact lenses. When a person attempts detox too early, it can make the autoimmune disease worse, and it can even lead to another autoimmune issue.

During a deep detox, if your gut and adrenals are impaired and you're lacking nutrients, the toxins jump ship from the organ where they live and head somewhere else. In my case, it was my eyelids, and it was miserable. I learned the hard way so you don't have to!

I recommend holding off on forceful detox protocols until you have finished the Fundamental Protocols and perhaps even the Advanced Protocols in this book.

- **Reduced sweating:** Most people with autoimmune thyroid disease have a reduced ability to sweat. While this is hardly a symptom most complain about, it is a symptom with many negative consequences, as sweating is a primary means to remove toxins from the body.
- **Acid and alkaline imbalance:** Most people who eat a standard American diet tend to have acidic bodies. This leads to a reduced output of some toxins from our urine. Luckily, there is a hack for that in this very chapter.

While in some cases, the extreme measures found in forceful

detoxes may need to be utilized, I've found that following the Liver Support Protocol can often recover a person's health in a safer and gentler way. Furthermore, people who have been strengthened using this protocol are going to have a better chance of tolerating not just the Advanced Protocols in this book but also more aggressive detox methods, if they are still needed later.

Before we go into exactly what the Liver Support Protocol entails, let's explore the role of toxins in Hashimoto's and where you are exposed to them in your daily life. It's pretty hard to eliminate toxins from your life if you don't know where to look for them! You should know that I've done extensive research in this area and therefore have a lot of information to share with you on the many potential toxins you have been or are being exposed to. Keep in mind that you don't have to become an expert yourself and you can take in as much or as little of this information as you'd like. You can also skip directly to the protocol if you're eager to get started (turn to page 110).

Toxic Exposure and Hashimoto's

The rates of Hashimoto's have been increasing worldwide over the last few decades, and some researchers are now saying up to 28 percent of the population may be affected (up to 37 percent in Italy!). In the last chapter, I discussed how improved diagnostic methods, such as cytology, are finding Hashimoto's more often. However, this does not fully account for the dramatic rise in Hashimoto's cases worldwide.

Numerous studies comparing thyroid tissues and blood samples taken from people during previous years have found that the incidence of Hashimoto's seems to be increasing worldwide. I believe that toxins are at least partially to blame, especially considering that areas with greater environmental toxicity and pollution have higher rates of Hashimoto's. Here are just two examples that illustrate my point:

- A 2003 review in *Thyroid* journal of the implications of radiation on autoimmune thyroid disease found that even though they were otherwise genetically and culturally similar, 81 percent of children who lived in a contaminated region of Ukraine after the 1986 Chernobyl nuclear disaster had thyroid antibodies, compared to only 17 percent of children living in another part of Ukraine that was farther from the nuclear disaster.

- A 2015 study in Sicily found that people living closer to a petrochemical complex, and thus subject to its pollution, were more likely to have a greater frequency of Hashimoto's and thyroid nodules.

While some thyroid researchers keep finding more and more genes that lead to autoimmune development, I personally think that we need to focus less on genes and more on our environment. After all, we can't change our genes, but we can change our environment, and new research in the field of epigenetics is now showing that environmental factors can determine the expression of genes.

Toxins are very much the elephant in the room that most conventional medical doctors do not address. For some people, a toxic exposure can bring on autoimmune thyroid disease as an initial trigger. Let's look at some of the toxins that could be triggering or exacerbating Hashimoto's.

Sick Building Syndrome

Have you ever walked into a building and just felt off? *Sick building syndrome* is a recently coined term to describe a collection of health symptoms experienced by one or more people due to exposure and time spent within a specific building.

This is due to poor indoor air quality that may be caused by various airborne toxins, such as off-gassing building materials, volatile organic compounds (VOCs), air pathogens, pollens, or molds. This is usually combined with faulty heating, air-conditioning, and ventilation systems—up to 30 percent of buildings may be affected!

People who work or live inside these buildings often have numerous nonspecific complaints such as skin symptoms, irritated mucous membranes, asthma symptoms, sensitivities, gut issues, headaches, fatigue, and irritability. The symptoms increase with stress and more time spent inside the building.

Mold

Mold in itself can be a powerful trigger for many autoimmune conditions, including autoimmune thyroid disease, asthma, and allergies. Mold does not necessarily cause Hashimoto's—rather, it pulls the trigger of a loaded genetic predisposition. This is important to note, as it depends on the person's genetic predisposition as to which type of autoimmune condition they will develop.

It's not uncommon to see a variety of symptoms within a family sharing the same home. For example, a family of four living in a moldy home may look like this:

- Mother with Hashimoto's
- Father with allergies and weight problems
- One child with asthma
- One child seemingly unaffected

If your symptoms started around the time that you moved into your home, there's a high potential that mold or toxic exposure may be the root cause of your condition. Potential symptoms can include elevated cholesterol, brain fog despite thyroid medications, and not getting well despite good nutrition. There are other signs related to mold that I have found in my clients:

- Living in a home with a basement that has flooded
- A stale, moldy smell in your home
- Multiple family members with varying levels of immune-related diseases

If mold is your root cause, doing all of the interventions in this book will be really helpful for you, but you will also need to move out of your toxic environment and do advanced mold protocols.

Everyday Toxins

While some people may have significant toxic exposures from known toxins, for others, the poisoning is much more subtle and results from accumulation due to exposure to chemicals in everyday life. Most people, even doctors, are unaware of the health implications of these chemicals. Here's a list of some of the most common toxins that have been recognized as endocrine disruptors and have been connected to altered hormone function and autoimmune disease. Please note, this list is not all exhaustive, and you may have additional unique toxic triggers. The following chemicals may affect thyroid activity directly, mimic other hormones, or affect the gut microbiome and immune system activity by various mechanisms:

- **Xenoestrogens:** Xenoestrogens are chemicals that mimic the effect of estrogen. As estrogen increases our need for thyroid hormone, it's possible that exposure to these chemicals may increase TSH, resulting in a triggering of the autoimmune process. Xenoestrogens include a variety of substances like soy, BPA, phthalates, and parabens found in foods, plastics, and personal care products.
- **Triclosan:** A common chemical, triclosan is found in antibacterial soaps, deodorants, hair sprays, and toothpastes. The structure of triclosan resembles the structure of thyroid hormones and has been associated with altered levels of thyroid hormone in animals. In fact, this ingredient has recently been banned by the FDA due to thyroid toxicity.
- **Bisphenol A (BPA):** BPA is found in plastics such as containers, baby formula cans, and even in the coating of store register receipts. It has been linked to cancers as well as reproductive disorders and developmental disorders. BPA also antagonizes

T3 receptors, essentially shutting them down. Rats exposed to BPA showed a long-term disruption of intestinal immune function. They were more likely to develop gut infections and more likely to suffer from food intolerance.

- **Heavy metals and metalloids:** These can be found in foods, personal care products, supplements, and home goods. A study of 1,587 people done by the National Health and Nutrition Examination Survey showed alterations in thyroid function in people who had shown exposure to metals in blood (lead, cadmium, and mercury) and urine (lead, cadmium, mercury, barium, cobalt, cesium, molybdenum, antimony, thallium, tungsten, and uranium). Copper is considered a less toxic heavy metal but has been associated with sabotaging thyroid function, as has the metalloid arsenic.
- **Halogens and halogen-containing chemicals:** These chemicals include bromide, chloride, and fluoride; are structurally similar to iodine; and may take up receptor sites in the thyroid gland. Unfortunately, their presence in the thyroid gland can lead to thyroid cell death and inflammation. Individuals exposed to high levels of halogen-containing substances have been found to have higher rates of thyroid antibodies.
  - ○ **Chlorine:** When found in polychlorinated biphenyls (PCBs), chlorine has been shown to be toxic to thyroid cells and to promote the onset of Hashimoto's through increasing TSH, thyroid antibodies, and thyroid size. PCBs are found in industrial products. Chlorine is also found in water systems, pools, cleaning products, and plastics.
  - ○ **Bromide:** This can be found in baked goods, plastics, soft drinks, and even our mattresses, which are coated with brominated flame retardants. Studies show bromine-containing substances—polybrominated diphenyl ethers (PBDEs)—are connected to an increased incidence of Hashimoto's.
  - ○ **Fluoride:** This thyroid-suppressing halogen is found in water, toothpaste, and some medications as well as in black,

green, and red tea. Using a reverse osmosis filter is the best way to get rid of fluoride.

- **Lithium:** When used as a medication, lithium has a long-known suppressive effect on the thyroid gland. Lithium is found in varied amounts in our drinking water, and the amounts found in water can increase TSH and lower free thyroid hormones.

Root Cause Research Corner: Fluoride Conspiracy

Most people know that fluoride has been added to the water supplies of most U.S. cities and some cities in the UK starting in the 1950s as a public health measure meant to prevent dental decay. However, most people don't know that fluoride was used as an antithyroid drug that suppressed thyroid activity in people with overactive thyroids *before* the invention of antithyroid drugs.

A dose of 2 to 5 mg per day was typically found to be effective for suppressing an overactive thyroid. If you're drinking eight cups of water each day, chances are, you are taking in enough fluoride to suppress your thyroid if you live in the typical fluoridated community!

While most Westernized countries have rightfully rejected fluoridation without any apparent consequences on tooth decay, the United States, Canada, and parts of the UK continue to fluoridate their water.

In research that was way overdue, a 2015 British study reported that medical practices in a fluoridated area of the UK (West Midlands vs. those in a nonfluoridated area, Greater Manchester) were *twice* as likely to report a high prevalence of hypothyroidism in their patients! Furthermore, analysis of different parts of the UK found that the rates of hypothyroidism were statistically matched to the rates of fluoride in the local water supply!

Radiation

A significant connection between radiation and thyroid autoimmunity has been found in people exposed to the nuclear disaster in Chernobyl. Recent studies have shown that even low doses of radiation can influence the immune system, possibly exacerbating certain autoimmune conditions such as asthma and Hashimoto's. One such study, conducted by Dr. Noriko Shimura at Ohu University in Japan, found that mice exposed to low doses of radiation had higher rates of autoimmune thyroid disease and overall higher numbers of thyroid antibodies.

Personal Care Products

Examining an average American woman's bathroom, you will likely find close to one hundred personal care products, including nail polish, lotion, shampoo, makeup remover, eyeliner, face masks, hairspray, perfume … the list goes on and on.

These products are full of chemicals that have not undergone safety studies to prove that they are not toxic. Most cosmetic chemists only test the chemicals on themselves to see if the products make them more aesthetically appealing. Conducting laboratory tests to assess blood levels and changes in organ or immune system function, or any other available medical tests for that matter, are not common practices followed by the cosmetic industry.

Women on average use twelve personal care and cosmetics products per day, which amounts to approximately 168 different chemical ingredients! In contrast, men use an average of six personal care products, or an average of eighty-five chemicals, on a daily basis.

However, many people don't realize that what we put on our skin eventually ends up circulating in our bodies. Often the topical application route actually ends up with us absorbing more of the toxin than we would have by swallowing it. This is because when we swallow a substance, our gut and liver process it first before it goes into the circulation system. When you apply substances through the skin, the substances skip the gatekeepers of the digestive tract and liver.

I Was Poisoned by Lip Gloss!

I didn't fully understand the toxins contained in makeup until in the summer of 2014, when I was personally poisoned by lip gloss.

In 2014, after almost two years of having my Hashimoto's in remission, I started to see a decline in my health. I was out of breath, began to have mood swings, felt fatigued, started losing my hair, and had tingling in my hands and feet. I was found to be anemic, and my TSH was around 4 μIU/mL (it had been around 1 μIU/mL the previous two years). For the first time in two years, instead of reducing the dose of my thyroid medication, I had to increase it.

I was suspicious that my symptoms felt a lot like heavy metal toxicity, so I tested my urine for heavy metals through ZRT Laboratory. Sure enough, tests revealed that I had a urinary arsenic level of 810 mcg/g Cr, while the normal level should be somewhere under 138 mcg/g Cr!

I dived into research mode and learned that arsenic can be found in soil, food, water, air, volcano ash, coal, pesticides, rice, chicken, chromated copper arsenate–treated wood, Ayurvedic supplements, and some makeup. I investigated every possible source, and then I remembered that the day after I began to use Benefit Benetint lip gloss, I woke up tired with a sore throat and swollen lymph nodes.

Arsenic can activate the Epstein-Barr virus, and my sore throat, fatigue, and swollen lymph nodes were due to waking up the dormant virus, which began to replicate in my thyroid gland.

Luckily, ditching the lip gloss, increasing my thyroid medications, and following the Fundamental Protocols eliminated all of my symptoms. However, I also needed the Advanced Protocols, including treatment for the Epstein-Barr virus, adrenals, and toxins to get back into remission again. Even after getting into remission, you might be faced with health challenges like I was. I hope that this book will be a guide for you to refer back to if that should ever happen.

I had been applying this lip gloss multiple times each day, unknowingly poisoning myself with each application. My heart aches when I begin to think about how many women are inadvertently poisoning themselves the same way. The lesson: pay attention to your personal care products!

A subset of pharmacology is dedicated to the study of pharmacokinetics and how different administration routes can impact the amount of a substance that goes into the body's circulation. The oral route of administration will result in the smallest amount of the substance moving into circulation, while alternative routes like rectal, vaginal, intravenous, intramuscular, inhalation, sublingual, and transdermal get directly into circulation.

The Environmental Working Group has found 146 cosmetic ingredients that may contain toxic impurities, and reported that 80 percent of personal care items contain these ingredients.

While it's difficult to pinpoint the exact reasons why seven women develop Hashimoto's for every one man with the condition, perhaps the use of endocrine-disrupting chemicals may play a role. Men generally use fewer personal care products, so perhaps women's personal care routine is partly responsible for the disproportionate female predominance of thyroid and autoimmune conditions.

The use of lipstick, in particular, has been connected with the development of lupus, another autoimmune condition. Absorption of toxins from the lips is more likely than from other cosmetics because the lips are a mucous membrane and because we may inadvertently ingest the products by licking our lips. As lip gloss is reapplied often, we also have a higher likelihood for exposure to the toxins.

Cosmetics in general are particularly problematic with regard to heavy metal contamination. A May 2011 report from Environmental Defence Canada tested a total of forty-nine pieces of makeup from six Canadian women for heavy metals and found some startling results! The majority of the tested products contained nickel (100 percent), lead (96 percent), beryllium (90 percent), and thallium (61 percent). Furthermore, 51 percent contained cadmium, while 20 percent contained arsenic.

You can obtain the full report from www.environmentaldefence. ca to see the comprehensive details and products tested. But just in case you think that only cheap or foreign products are the issue, I want to share that popular and expensive brands like Clinique, Sephora, L'Oréal, and MAC were all found to have these heavy metals.

Additionally, the popular Benefit Benetint lip gloss had the most heavy metals, including arsenic, beryllium, cadmium, nickel, lead, and thallium. The lip gloss was found to have 70 ppm of arsenic, while the maximum acceptable allowance of arsenic in food is <0.1 ppm, meaning the lip gloss contained 700 times the amount of arsenic that would be reported to be toxic in food. While we obviously eat more food than lip gloss, due to the porous nature of our lips, the arsenic from the lip gloss can be absorbed more readily than it would if it were eaten. Furthermore, 110 ppm of lead, or ten times the allowable amount in food, was found in the product.

I found this out the hard way, so hopefully you won't have to!

Cleaning Products

Conventional cleaning supplies used to clean our bathrooms, kitchens, and floors are full of toxic chemicals. You can make your own cleaning supplies or purchase ones made from natural ingredients. The Environmental Working Group also has a database of safer, cleaner alternatives (www.ewg.org/guides/cleaners).

Cooking Utensils

Metals like aluminum and nickel can leach into our bodies from cookware and cooking utensils, especially when the utensils are heated up. While stainless steel pans have been considered a healthier alternative to Teflon-coated pans, nickel from the stainless steel pans can be problematic for some.

Food Pharmacology

Over the course of this book, you will come to learn that food can be used as medicine and that food can also be toxic! The Root Cause Intro Diet is two pronged—it focuses on reducing toxic foods and adding more healing foods.

Food toxins can be substances that are found on foods (such as pesticides, the residue of which can contribute to overall toxic load) and in foods (such as mercury, which is known to disrupt thyroid function and which you might ingest when you eat certain types of fish, especially tuna). I'm also referring to certain foods themselves, which have a structural makeup that can trigger a toxic reaction in people with Hashimoto's and other autoimmune conditions.

People with Hashimoto's may also have a toxic reaction to foods due to their structural makeup. Genetically modified foods in particular have been implicated in triggering immune-related health problems because of the presence of foreign DNA from viruses and bacteria used to modify the foods. Furthermore, difficult-to-digest food proteins, such as gluten, dairy, and soy proteins, can cause and perpetuate an autoimmune response due to molecular mimicry. If you have intestinal permeability (always a precursor to autoimmune disease), your body is more likely to recognize these proteins as foreign invaders and make antibodies to them. When this happens, you can develop a food toxicity reaction known as a food sensitivity. Food sensitivities are different from allergies in that they are produced by the IgG and IgA branch of the immune system, whereas food allergies are mediated by the IgE branch of the immune system.

Chernobyl Child

The more I learn about the many triggers of Hashimoto's and look back on my personal health history, the more I've come to realize that my condition likely started developing decades before I was officially diagnosed and perhaps fifteen years before my obvious symptoms began. I grew up in Hostynne, Poland, a small farming village on the southeast side of Poland, and was exposed to radiation from Chernobyl at age four. My mom recalls that I was a child prone to anxiety, and I can't think of a time when I didn't have cold hands and feet!

I've already mentioned the startling statistic—as many as 81 percent of children exposed to Chernobyl had thyroid antibodies! Once thyroid antibodies are present, a person will have a fluctuation of thyroid hormone levels that lasts for decades before hypothyroidism develops. This fluctuation can cause many confusing symptoms, often of both hypothyroidism and hyperthyroidism. This was the case for me, and likely the root cause of my bouts of anxiety, depression, cold hands, and poor growth during childhood and young adulthood. Whether you've been exposed to radiation or another toxin, I want you to know that recovering your health is possible!

Food sensitivities and food allergies aren't just different because of their distinct immune system affiliation; they also produce different reactions through different time frames. A food sensitivity will produce symptoms such as irritable bowel symptoms, headaches, and skin breakouts, which may take up to four days to manifest (referred to as type IV delayed hypersensitivity), while an allergic reaction is likely to be much more severe and immediate (referred to as a type I hypersensitivity).

Food sensitivities and thyroid antibodies, specifically TPO and TG antibodies, are both moderated by the IgG branch of the immune system, which could have something to do with the fact that Hashimoto's and food sensitivities often co-occur. It's interesting to note that both food sensitivity reactions and the autoimmune response seen in Hashimoto's are type IV delayed hypersensitivity reactions. In my experience with clients, eating foods that stimulate the release of the IgG antibodies and promote a type IV response will also increase thyroid antibodies and an immune response against the thyroid. Perhaps it's a turning-on-the-faucet effect, or perhaps these proteins cross-react with the thyroid gland. More research is needed to quantify the exact reaction, but I can say that most people with Hashimoto's (up to 88 percent of my clients and readers) will have a reduction in thyroid symptoms and antibodies after removing reactive food proteins.

Circulating immune complexes (CICs), which are made up of an antibody and the reactive food protein, are produced in autoimmune disease whenever a reactive food is eaten, and the CICs accumulate in the liver, leading to impaired liver function.

Let's take a closer look at the most common trigger for toxic reactions in people with Hashimoto's (and most other autoimmune diseases).

Gluten is a protein found in barley, rye, and wheat. It's a staple in the Western diet that you'll encounter in most breads, cereals, and pasta. Gluten-containing foods can create a toxic response in people with autoimmune disease, including those with Hashimoto's. The most severe form of gluten response is seen in people with celiac disease.

An autoimmune attack on the intestines occurs when someone with celiac disease eats gluten, and this attack leads to a destruction of the villi, which are delicate, hairlike projections that cover the intestines and help to digest and absorb nutrients from food. This damage of the villi causes people with celiac disease to become malnourished, no matter how much food they eat, because the body is not able to absorb the nutrients from the food that is consumed.

Symptoms may vary from person to person. Some people may have terrible diarrhea, others constipation, nausea, vomiting, acid reflux, weight loss, easy bruising, anemia, depression, hair loss, or infertility. Many of these symptoms mimic those of other diseases, which is why celiac disease has been called the great imitator. This is also why celiac disease can often go undiagnosed for so long, as it is often mistaken for other issues. Left undetected, people with celiac disease are more likely to develop intestinal cancer. Even tiny amounts of gluten can cause extreme gut distress and other severe symptoms.

Celiac disease can also co-occur with other autoimmune disorders, including lupus, Addison's disease, and Hashimoto's. Studies have estimated that between 1.2 and 15 percent of Hashimoto's patients also have celiac disease. Additional research done in the Netherlands with 104 Hashimoto's patients found that 50 percent of them had celiac-specific genes. The same researchers also tested the inverse relationship—that is, the occurrence of Hashimoto's in people diagnosed with celiac disease, and they found that 18 percent of celiac patients also had Hashimoto's.

While gluten causes intestinal permeability in most people, celiac disease antibodies can also cross-react with thyroid antibodies, and this may be one of the reasons for the common co-occurrence. Up to 20 percent of people with celiac disease and Hashimoto's can get Hashimoto's into remission within a year of going gluten-free, and some may go into remission in as little as three months.

When Italian researchers placed people with subclinical hypothyroidism and celiac disease on a gluten-free diet, thyroid function normalized in a significant percentage of them. Take a look at these specific findings:

- In 71 percent of people who strictly followed a one-year gluten withdrawal, there was a normalization of subclinical hypothyroidism.
- Another 19 percent of people who followed the gluten-free diet were able to normalize their thyroid antibodies. "In distinct

cases, gluten withdrawal may single-handedly reverse the abnormality," the researchers concluded.

Some new research suggests that people with autoimmune conditions may have non-celiac gluten sensitivity (NCGS), a newly described condition in which people have celiac-like reactions to gluten but don't test positive to the celiac antibodies nor do they present the characteristic damage to intestinal cells observed with celiac disease. Other than symptoms, there is not a specific test for NCGS, but a 2002 study in the *European Journal of Endocrinology* found that 43 percent of people with Hashimoto's showed activated mucosal T cell immunity, which is usually correlated with gluten sensitivity.

What's the connection between celiac disease, gluten sensitivity, and autoimmune diseases such as Hashimoto's? It's found in gluten's ability to cause intestinal permeability. When gluten proteins cause damage to the intestinal wall, gaps can form, creating a leaky gut that allows food particles to enter into the bloodstream. Once in the gut, these particles are recognized as foreign substances by the immune system, and the body launches an immune attack every time those foods are eaten. The leaky gut reaction to gluten is thought to be a spectrum. In most healthy individuals, gluten causes a small degree of intestinal permeability that is short lasting (minutes), while in those with celiac disease, the reaction can be more severe and last numerous days. In NCGS, the reaction will be somewhere in the middle.

This can make eating extremely difficult and unpleasant, causing symptoms that may include diarrhea, heartburn, upset stomach, pain, and nerve tingling. Intestinal permeability has been linked to other autoimmune conditions, and people with celiac disease are at risk of developing those as well—especially if they don't change their diet.

There is a strong connection between gluten reactions and the thyroid. Some people will be able to completely put their conditions into remission by going gluten-free, while others may need to dig a bit deeper (as in my case). The majority will feel exponentially better! In my client work, as well as my survey of 2,232 people with Hashimoto's, roughly 88 percent of people with Hashimoto's feel significantly better gluten-free! Given the strong connection between gluten reactions and the thyroid, this is not surprising.

The results among my readers and clients have been so profound that I recommend that everyone with Hashimoto's eliminate gluten for two weeks to gauge if they see an improvement in symptoms.

Here's a short sampling from readers and clients who have gone gluten-free:

- "Gluten-free diet has helped me reduce antibodies almost to a normal range."
- "Going gluten-free helped me tremendously. It took eight months to feel the difference, and now after two years, most of my symptoms are gone. Nothing to lose by going gluten-free."
- "Since I went gluten-free, my hair started growing back, my bloating and diarrhea have gone, no more reflux either."
- "Going gluten-free has helped my hair to start growing back after losing all my hair—even my eyebrows and eyelashes."
- "Gluten-free and soy-free for three months and I was able to lower my meds, and [my] stomach pain, alternating diarrhea and constipation, anxiety, and body aches [are] all gone!!"
- "I'm gluten-free and have brought my antibodies down to normal range. So thankful!"

Some people (myself included) will have to dig a bit deeper than gluten to achieve remission, though. My personal experience, extensive research, and client assessments have revealed that it's not just gluten that can be a toxic food for Hashimoto's. The most common food sensitivities in Hashimoto's are to gluten, dairy (this was my biggest one), soy, eggs, sugar, grains (especially corn), nightshades (potatoes, tomatoes, eggplants, and peppers), caffeine, alcohol, and nuts and seeds.

Many of my readers and clients have experienced noticeable benefits from removing these foods too: 88 percent reported feeling better gluten-free; 87 percent reported feeling better on a sugar-free diet; 81 percent reported feeling better on a grain-free or Paleo diet; 79 percent reported feeling better on a dairy-free diet, 63 percent or so said they felt better soy-free; and egg- and nightshade-free diets were helpful to 47 percent and 48 percent of those surveyed, respectively. Another 15 percent of people saw improvement with a nut-free diet, while 7 percent reported feeling better off seeds. The autoimmune Paleo diet, which excludes all of the above listed foods, helped 75 percent of people feel better. If you already know that you react to the above-mentioned foods, you can remove them from your diet immediately. Otherwise, we will gradually eliminate them from your diet in the Fundamental Adrenal Recovery and Gut Balance Protocols and gauge improvement.

Food Research

While I have seen tremendous improvements in my health, as well as the health of my clients, through eliminating reactive foods, the research supporting the use of nutrition for Hashimoto's is severely lacking (with the exception of co-occurring celiac disease and Hashimoto's). This remains true years after I wrote my first book and then spent a great deal of time spreading awareness about the role of food with Hashimoto's. I thought for sure that a research center would try out the various methods I found to be helpful, but that never happened. However, two years later, I realized that I didn't have to wait for a research center—I could do my own research with the help of my Root Cause Rebel community (or maybe that I *had* to do it!).

I conducted a survey of my readers from May 10, 2015, to May 31, 2015. In total, 2,232 people answered the survey, 1,991 of whom reported to have Hashimoto's. Only seventy-eight (3.5 percent) were also diagnosed with celiac disease. It should be noted that this method of conducting research has limitations by traditional research standards: it was directed at a biased group (they were all my educated readers, after all!), and I did not have a control group. Nonetheless, it revealed a lot of exciting trends, mirroring the same patterns I've seen in my private clients but in a much larger sample size. If you trust people who are just like you, then you will find this information helpful.

I asked the readers to specify the foods that they believed to be reactive for them as well as the body system where they experienced their symptoms. For example, they were to categorize symptoms such as postnasal drip, congestion, cough, and asthma-related symptoms under *Lungs*. Symptoms of constipation, diarrhea, cramping, bloating, nausea, gas, acid reflux, burning, and burping were labeled as *Gut*. Here are the symptoms and body systems they could select based on their experience:

COMMON FOOD REACTIONS

Body System	Symptoms
Lungs	Postnasal drip, congestion, cough, asthma
Gut	Constipation, diarrhea, cramping, bloating, nausea, gas, acid reflux, burning, burping
Heart	Increased pulse, palpitations
Skin	Acne, eczema, itchiness
Muscles	Joint aches, pain, swelling, tingling, numbness
Brain	Headache, dizziness, brain fog, anxiety, depression, fatigue, insomnia

The results revealed a great deal about the foods that Hashimoto's patients are sensitive to. Out of all of the surveyed people, 76 percent reported being sensitive to gluten, 64 percent to sugar, 57 percent to dairy, 44 percent to grains, 42 percent to caffeine, 41 percent to soy, 33 percent to corn, 19 percent to nightshades, 18 percent to eggs, 15 percent to nuts, 12 percent to red meat, 11 percent to cruciferous vegetables, 9 percent to fruit, and 7 percent to seeds.

The majority of reactions, with the exception of those that were triggered by sugar and caffeine, manifested in the gut domain. Symptoms included constipation, diarrhea, cramping, bloating, nausea, gas, acid reflux, burning, and burping. Sugar resulted primarily in brain-related symptoms such as headaches, dizziness, brain fog, anxiety, depression, fatigue, and insomnia, although the gut domain was also affected. As expected, caffeine was associated with increased pulse and palpitations (heart) and greater feelings of anxiety. Nightshade vegetables were associated with joint aches, pain, swelling, tingling, and numbness. Nuts and fruit were associated with skin reactions including acne, eczema, and itchiness.

The second most common domain impacted was the brain, which was reported to be affected by reactions to gluten, caffeine, soy, corn, eggs, cruciferous vegetables, and seeds.

In parallel with my clinical observations, dairy was implicated in postnasal drip, congestion, cough, and asthma-related symptoms. Surprisingly, red meat was implicated in the muscle domain as well.

Out of the 1,736 of the surveyed Hashimoto's patients who tried a gluten-free diet, 80 percent reported seeing an improvement in their digestive symptoms, while 13 percent did not report improvement. The rest did not have any digestive symptoms before going gluten-free.

FOOD REACTIONS IN HASHIMOTO'S PATIENTS

The survey respondents were asked whether a food was reactive for them and where the reaction was seen in their bodies.

Food	Percentage That Reported Sensitivity	Most Common Symptom Domain	Second Most Common Symptom Domain
Gluten	76	Gut (57%)	Brain (41%)
Sugar	64	Brain (35%)	Gut (25%)
Dairy	57	Gut (44%)	Lungs (21%)
Grains	44	Gut (30%)	Brain (17%)

Food	Percentage That Reported Sensitivity	Most Common Symptom Domain	Second Most Common Symptom Domain
Caffeine	42	Heart (27%)	Brain (18%)
Soy	41	Gut (16%)	Brain (9%)
Corn	33	Gut (22%)	Brain (8%)
Nightshades	19	Gut (9%)	Muscles (7%)
Eggs	18	Gut (15%)	Brain (4%)
Nuts	15	Gut (12%)	Skin (4%)
Red Meat	12	Gut (11%)	Muscles (2%)
Cruciferous Vegetables	11	Gut (12%)	Brain (1%)
Fruit	9	Gut (8%)	Skin (3%)
Seeds	7	Gut (7%)	Brain (1%)

Testing for Celiac Disease and Food Sensitivities

Current testing for celiac disease is far from perfect, with the blood-screening test often coming back negative in all but the most advanced cases. However, if you do suspect celiac disease, you might consider completing a genetic test with a company such as 23andMe to help determine whether you're genetically at risk to develop celiac disease.

Tests for food sensitivities, such as gluten sensitivity, are even less reliable. This is why the best and cheapest approach is to eliminate gluten and other wheat-containing products for at least three weeks, watch for improvement, and if unsure, reintroduce to check for reactions.

If you do use this elimination approach, it's important to remember that healing takes time. A gluten-free diet is necessary to heal the intestines, and while some improvements may be immediate, complete symptom resolution can take from three months to two years of following a strict gluten-free diet. Even a small amount of gluten can cause a huge setback, and you may discover that you need to eliminate other foods as well to experience complete healing. You'll discover the complete list of foods to remove in the first step of the protocol. But first let's look at the protocol overview.

The Two-Week Liver Support Protocol

Now it's time to get into the specifics of the protocol. Here are the four steps:

1. Remove potentially triggering foods.
2. Add supportive foods.
3. Reduce toxic exposure.
4. Support detox pathways.

Symptom improvement occurs rapidly because as triggers are removed and nutrient deficiencies are addressed, the liver is able to clear out toxins and process hormones more efficiently.

People with thyroid disease will also begin to feel better because as more of the liver enzymes are freed up to work on hormones instead of toxins, the body has more access to T3, the active thyroid hormone.

The body produces the active T3 hormone through a conversion process from either endogenous T4 that's produced in the body or exogenous T4 that is taken as a medication. What this means in very simple terms is that with a healthy liver, our bodies can utilize our own thyroid hormones as well as our thyroid medication much more efficiently.

I now start all of my clients on this Liver Support Protocol before we start addressing their adrenals, gut, food, medications, digestion, nutrient deficiencies, and infections. And definitely way before they start going into forced detox protocols! Even though toxins may be a significant root cause for many with Hashimoto's, it's important to remember that the toxins should be ushered out of the body gently and slowly so they don't do damage on their way out.

Once we support the liver, you will be able to tolerate additional lifestyle changes and supplements much better. Are you ready to get started?

During this two-week protocol, I'd like to introduce you to the Root Cause Intro Diet. As you'll come to learn, nutrition is a major part of healing! In fact, nutrition is so important, it takes up two steps of the protocol!

Step 1: Remove Potentially Triggering Foods

You're going to cut out gluten, dairy, sugar, soy, caffeine, and alcohol. Eliminating processed foods will help you a great deal in removing these triggers foods. If you've already removed most of these foods and additional reactive foods from your life, continue your current exclusion and focus on incorporating more supportive foods (step 2), reducing toxic exposure (step 3), and supporting detox pathways (step 4).

Gluten

Gluten must be completely avoided for healing and relief of symptoms; there is no such thing as partially gluten-free. In order to completely cut gluten from your diet, you will need to remove all items containing wheat, barley, and rye. This is harder than it sounds, as many processed foods contain some form of gluten as a stabilizing agent. Even foods you might assume are safe, such as salad dressings, marinades, barbecue sauces, and soups, should be checked for sources of gluten.

If you have celiac disease, you could notice an improvement in symptoms within a few days, although it will take three months to two years for full healing. In those with gluten sensitivity, improvement should be seen in two to three weeks, and healing within six to eight weeks. There is some preliminary evidence that celiac disease is permanent, while gluten intolerance, on the other hand, may be reversible. Thus a person with celiac disease will require lifelong strict avoidance of gluten, while a person with gluten intolerance may be able to recover from gluten-related reactions.

DAIRY REPLACEMENTS

Dairy Type	Replacement Options
Milk	Coconut milk, almond milk, cashew milk
Butter	Coconut oil, ghee
Yogurt	Coconut yogurt, almond yogurt
Whey protein	Pea protein, hydrolyzed beef protein, egg white protein*
Ice cream	Coconut ice cream, almond ice cream, or pureed frozen bananas
Cheese	Cashew and other nut cheeses; dairy-free, soy-free cheeses like the brand Daiya

*Likely to cause an adverse reaction with long-term use

Dairy

Dairy is another common reactive food in people with Hashimoto's. Some people may have a primary dairy sensitivity, while others may develop a secondary dairy sensitivity due to the gluten-induced damage to the gut.

You may have heard of lactose intolerance, a lack of enzymes that prevents proper breakdown of the milk sugar lactose. This is just one type of dairy reaction, but it is not the same as dairy sensitivity, which, like gluten sensitivity, is mediated by the immune system.

People with Hashimoto's usually have sensitivities to the proteins found in dairy: casein and whey. All cow milk products including milk, cheese, yogurt, ice cream, and even butter should be avoided. "Healthy" protein powders containing whey protein also need to be eliminated. Some nondairy cheeses may contain casein, the most problematic of the dairy proteins. Processed foods may contain dairy proteins and are best avoided.

Please note, although dairy products are kept in the same part of the grocery store as eggs, eggs are not considered dairy.

Safe Protein Powders

Most protein powders on the market contain soy and dairy, which are two very reactive proteins for people with Hashimoto's. Egg white proteins are less reactive, but unfortunately those with Hashimoto's who start using them often find themselves with new onset egg reactions because egg whites are difficult to digest for people with intestinal permeability. The protein powders that are the best tolerated by people with Hashimoto's are pea protein and hydrolyzed beef protein. Both are hypoallergenic and easy to digest. I recommend using the pea protein for cleansing (Liver Support Protocol) and the hydrolyzed beef protein for building (Adrenal Recovery and Gut Balance Protocols). Hydrolyzed beef protein offers a special advantage, as it is less likely to cause new food reactions due to the hydrolysis process, which breaks the protein into tiny pieces. Surprisingly, hydrolyzed beef protein is very tasty. It doesn't taste like beef but has a slight milky taste. I've developed the Rootcology AI Paleo Protein to contain hydrolyzed beef protein that is free of any fillers and compliant with even the strictest autoimmune protocol as well as the Rootcology Organic Pea Protein to be used for cleansing.

If you're not experiencing full relief from the gluten-free diet, dairy avoidance may be needed for three to six months. Many people regain their ability to tolerate dairy after six months, but some will need to avoid it indefinitely.

Sugar

In addition to table sugar, avoiding processed foods that contain sugar or high fructose corn syrup as an ingredient will be important during the Liver Support Protocol. You can use stevia, Truvia, Xylitol, or

Root Cause Research Corner: Not-So-Sweet Sweeteners

NutraSweet, Equal (aspartame), and Splenda (sucralose) have been connected to Hashimoto's. Dr. Isaac Sachmechi, a professor at Mount Sinai, reported that two of his patients saw a complete remission of Hashimoto's after quitting artificial sweeteners. This was the only change they made! If you haven't already done so, I recommend removing these from your diet permanently.

trehalose as an alternative, but steer clear of sucralose (Splenda) or saccharine, as they have both been implicated in triggering Hashimoto's.

Soy

Many gluten-free products contain soy, which can be problematic for thyroid patients and can worsen the autoimmune attack on the thyroid. I believe that my thyroid condition became worse after eating soy-containing gluten-free products. After one month off soy products, my thyroid antibodies dropped from 800 IU/mL to 380 IU/mL.

You will want to avoid edamame beans, soy milk, tofu, tempeh, miso, and soy sauce. Additionally, you will want to eliminate processed foods and supplements, which often contain soy-based ingredients. This includes vegetarian and vegan products, which can include soy lecithin, bean curd, hydrolyzed soy protein, or hydrolyzed vegetable protein. If you see any of these listed on a product label, put it back!

Caffeine

While coffee and tea have numerous health benefits, and coffee can actually be helpful for liver disease, we are going to temporarily remove caffeine products during the Fundamental Protocols.

Caffeine in coffee and tea can prevent us from resting when we should, and this can put our bodies in a fight-or-flight setting instead of a rest-and-digest setting. Caffeine is known to interfere with sleep, and because most of our liver detoxifying and healing takes place when we're sleeping, we want to avoid anything that may interfere with sleep. We want to give the body every opportunity to heal. Additionally, caffeine weakens the adrenals and can increase gut permeability. Furthermore, tea is problematic because of fluoride content, while coffee has the potential to contain mold or cross-react with gluten.

If you've been drinking caffeine for a while, you may want to wean yourself off instead of going cold turkey, as caffeine is an addictive substance. Reducing your intake by 50 percent every day can be helpful. For example, if you usually drink two cups of coffee per day, dropping down to one cup, then a half cup, a quarter cup, and then discontinuing may be a gentler process.

You still may get withdrawal headaches. Magnesium supplements, Epsom salt baths, hot lemon water, and herbal coffee substitutes like Dandy Blend can help in the transition period.

Instead of caffeine, you can have the following:

- **Hot lemon water:** Drinking this first thing in the morning and throughout the day will wake you up better than any tea or coffee and will help support your stomach acid and your liver's detox pathways.
- **Maca latte:** The adaptogen maca will support your adrenals and hormones, while the coconut milk will help your blood sugar stay stable throughout the day. Bonus: this tastes like a latte (see page 129)!
- **Green juice:** This will give you plenty of nutrients and energy in a broken-down, usable form.
- **Turmeric tea:** A great replacement for hot tea, turmeric tea is an excellent and delicious way to detox (see page 124).

- **Mint tea:** This is a simple and delicious herbal tea. As a bonus, mint also suppresses SIBO, a common Hashimoto's imbalance.
- **Dandy Blend:** Enjoy this gluten-free herbal mix that tastes like coffee.
- **Spa water:** Mix purified water with fruit for a fun way to quench your thirst.

I'd love to share more recipes with you; please go to www.thyroid pharmacist.com/action to grab them.

Alcohol

Alcohol leads to blood sugar imbalances, a liver backlog, leaky gut, and an overgrowth of bacteria in the small intestine. Yes, even that "healthy" glass of wine too! If you miss the taste and feel of alcohol, you can replace alcohol with my Fermented Margarita or Virgin Mojito (see pages 129–130). The probiotics in the drinks will support your liver and gut.

So what can you eat? Step 2 will go into specific supportive foods you'll want to eat during the Liver Support Protocol, but generally speaking, you will want to focus on eating a nutrient-dense diet. This is a diet that includes different varieties and healthy portions of meat, all vegetables, all fruit, nuts, seeds, and eggs as long as you are not sensitive.

Step 2: Add Supportive Foods

I love using delicious foods to nourish and support the body back to health—this is truly using food as medicine! Here's a list of my recommended superfoods to incorporate into your daily routine during the two-week Liver Support Protocol (and hopefully you'll love and use them beyond). The superfoods are listed in order of importance. Try to commit to incorporating at least three or four of these into your routine. Bonus points if you can incorporate all eleven.

1. Hot lemon water: The cleansing properties in lemon juice support stomach and liver detoxification pathways. I recommend drinking hot lemon water alongside thyroid medication because the acidity

Suggestions for Dining Out During the Fundamental Protocols

Many restaurants have gluten-free menus, but eating out can still be challenging, as unless the entire restaurant is gluten-free, your gluten-free meal could still be cross-contaminated during preparation. Even a small amount of gluten can trigger a reaction (often manifesting as severe gastrointestinal symptoms). It's important to note that abstaining from gluten can unmask your gluten sensitivity, meaning that gluten exposure after a period of abstinence may trigger more acute symptoms than the chronic low-grade symptoms you had while eating gluten on a daily basis. This is because the absence of your trigger food will allow for reactive cells to build up, resulting in a stronger reaction when the food is introduced again in the body's effort to clear the toxin out.

Some foods more likely to be safe to order while you're dining out are the Cobb salad (greens, tomato, bacon, grilled chicken, boiled egg, onions, avocado, and cheese) or the Greek salad (greens, some variation of grilled chicken, olives, tomatoes, bell peppers, onions, cucumbers, and feta cheese). Be sure to ask the waiter for grilled chicken and to hold the cheese and dressing (many salad dressings have gluten, soy, and high fructose corn syrup). I recommend olive oil and lemon juice as a delicious alternative to dressing.

Grilled meats and steamed or grilled veggies are often an excellent option as well. To help prevent cross-contamination from breaded foods, you can ask that your food be grilled or steamed in foil.

You can get ahead of potential cross-contamination exposure by taking a supplement such as the Pure Encapsulations Gluten/Dairy Digest supplement. Though this product will not eliminate your reactions completely, it could possibly minimize adverse reactions.

from the lemon will aid in absorption. You can drink this instead of caffeine and you'll see a marked difference in your energy levels. A lot of people who drink this in the morning never go back to caffeine because they feel so much better! Drink it first thing in the morning on an empty stomach. Use the juice of one-half to one organic lemon in a cup of hot purified water. Add stevia or maple syrup to taste, if you'd like.

2. The Root Cause Green Smoothie: This green smoothie is packed with nutrition for your thyroid and can help detoxify and reduce inflammation. It combines a hypoallergenic protein source (pea) with fat from coconut milk and fiber from veggies.

As the smoothie is blended into tiny particles, it is much easier to digest compared to a regular breakfast, making the nutrients more readily available and creating more energy. Even though it's blended, remember to still chew the smoothie to help activate your digestive process. All of the ingredients have been chosen for a strategic reason:

- The coconut milk base is a hypoallergenic source of fat and can help reduce inflammation and stabilize blood sugar due to its good fat content.
- Adding an avocado increases the fat- and blood-sugar-stabilizing content, and gives the smoothie a pudding-like consistency.
- Veggies add fiber and micronutrients, which are more readily available due to using a blender to break the fiber and nutrients apart.
- Sea salt can help with supporting the adrenals, which are often stressed in people with Hashimoto's.

People who have tried the Root Cause Green Smoothie have said that it helps them feel less hungry, more relaxed and calm, and full of energy. If needed, you can even double the recipe to make enough for lunch!

Root Cause Green Smoothie

1 cup mixed baby greens

2 large carrots

1 ripe avocado

1 stick celery

1 cucumber

1 bunch basil leaves

1 cup coconut milk

1 scoop pea protein powder

Sea salt to taste

Combine all ingredients in a blender and blend until smooth.

Optional additions include one tablespoon of any of the following: camu powder (boosts vitamin C), cod liver oil (anti-inflammatory), coconut kefir probiotics, maca root powder (helps increase body temperature and stabilizes hormones), or turmeric powder (anti-inflammatory).

While most people who have tried the green smoothie love it, some people (ahem, my husband, Michael) may not like the pudding-like consistency and the warmth of the smoothie. To create a thinner, milk-like consistency and a "cold and tropical flavor"—as my husband describes his ideal smoothie—you can make the following adjustments:

- Skip the avocado and add a tablespoon of chia seeds instead. Chia seeds are a less creamy source of good fat.
- Add the juice of one lemon or lime to make it more tropical and to support digestive juices.
- Blend the contents with a cup of ice cubes to make the smoothie cold and give it a more milky consistency.

While the carrots and coconut naturally add sweetness, if you are coming off the standard American diet, you may want to initially add a boost of fruit, like a quarter cup of berries, half a banana, or half a green apple as your taste buds transition to appreciating the natural sweetness in coconuts and carrots.

3. Beets: Beets are rich in phytonutrients, have anti-inflammatory and antioxidant qualities, and support detoxification. Beets are an especially excellent food for people with the MTHFR gene mutation, as they are rich in folate and betaine, which help to break down homocysteine, giving people a natural adaptation to the gene mutation. Aim for one to two servings each week. As beets are naturally high in sugar, be sure to combine them with a healthy fat or protein source.

4. Cruciferous veggies: Crucifers contain nutrients that help support the liver's detoxification. These vegetables include cabbage, broccoli, cauliflower, kale, and turnips. I recommend buying organic, especially for kale because it tends to pick up a lot of toxins in the environment.

There's a myth that these vegetables aren't good for people with Hashimoto's, but this is not true. While cruciferous veggies do contain glucosinolates, which may block iodine absorption into the thyroid, most patients with Hashimoto's do not have an iodine deficiency, and the goitrogenic mechanism in these healthy vegetables should not be an issue. Plus, you'd have to eat a lot of them for the goitrogenic effect. Cruciferous vegetables are only truly goitrogenic in a raw state, so if you are concerned about your iodine levels, you can lightly steam or ferment them.

5. Cilantro: Cilantro is a natural chelator, which means it will bind to certain toxins and help excrete them from the body. Cilantro helps remove toxins in a gentle way and is delicious when added to salads, avocados, green juices, smoothies, and salsas. Please note that while chlorella and spirulina are also natural chelators, I do not routinely recommend these for people with Hashimoto's due to their high iodine content and their potential to modify the immune system.

Thyroid Myths: Cruciferous Vegetables

A common myth in the thyroid world is that goitrogens such as cruciferous vegetables should be avoided because they suppress thyroid function. Delicious and healthy vegetables like cabbage, Brussels sprouts, broccoli, kale, and cauliflower have gotten a bad rap due to some old nomenclature and outdated understanding of thyroid disease.

Goitrogen is a word that was coined in the 1950s to describe a substance that causes the formation of a goiter, also known as an enlarged thyroid gland. It's a very deceiving word and can mean a variety of different things for different substances, ranging from suppressing the release of thyroid hormone, to changing the way thyroid hormone is produced in the body, to suppressing the absorption of iodine.

Cruciferous vegetables have been identified as goitrogenic because they have the potential to block iodine absorption. This was a legitimate concern in the 1950s because during that time the primary reason for hypothyroidism was iodine deficiency and any further changes in iodine levels were potentially problematic.

Public efforts have since been made to add iodine to salt supplies in most industrialized countries, and Hashimoto's is now the primary reason for hypothyroidism, responsible for 90 to 97 percent of cases of hypothyroidism in the United States. Furthermore, iodine deficiency is not widespread in people with Hashimoto's.

Unless a person is otherwise sensitive to them, cruciferous vegetables are perfectly healthy for people with Hashimoto's and should not impact thyroid function. In the case that a person does have hypothyroidism due to iodine deficiency, they can still enjoy crucifers as long as they are cooked or fermented. Cooking and fermenting will break down the iodine-blocking components.

That said, some people may not tolerate broccoli, Brussels sprouts, and cauliflower. However, most reactions experienced by people with Hashimoto's will be due to their highly fermentable nature, which can exacerbate SIBO. Up to 50 percent of people with Hashimoto's may have SIBO (explored in detail in chapter 11). A small percentage of Hashimoto's patients may also have sulfur sensitivity, which may be exacerbated by crucifers—this will be explored in greater detail in the Advanced Protocols.

There is one goitrogen that I do always recommend avoiding with Hashimoto's and that's soy. Soy consumption has been linked with increased thyroid antibodies.

6. Fiber: Fiber aids our ability to excrete toxins and excess hormones. Most people can tolerate natural fiber found in fruits and veggies, but be careful with fiber in supplement forms (such as inulin, fructooligosaccharide [FOS], or psyllium supplements), as these can aggravate intestinal permeability and SIBO. If you haven't been in the habit of eating a lot of fiber, I recommend starting off slowly and gradually adding more to your diet.

7. Sprouts and seedlings: The sprouts and seedlings of plants have natural enzymes that break toxins apart. In the last few decades, the use of plant enzymes has been recognized as a helpful method for clearing toxins and endocrine disruptors from water. While most studies have been done outside of the human body, a study using a powder from broccoli sprouts found that the sprouts were able to enhance detoxification of airborne pollutants—this may be especially important for people living in big cities that have a lot of toxins.

Radish seedlings were shown to remove up to 88 percent of BPA, a thyroid-disrupting chemical found in plastics.

8. Greens juices and chlorophyll: Green juices are full of healing nutrients! Since they are in liquid form, they also make the nutrients easily digestible and accessible. In addition to the numerous vitamins they offer, green juices are also wonderful sources of chlorophyll, a green pigment contained in plants. Chlorophyll has been found to have various health benefits, including detoxification, reduced inflammation and oxidative stress, raised iron levels, and even natural deodorization by neutralizing odors. Juices are an excellent way to boost energy any time of day! Green juices should be primarily composed of vegetables with some fruit like green apples for flavor. Using a specialized juicer, known as a masticating juicer that "chews" the vegetables instead of cutting them, you can make yourself a batch of juice that can be sipped all day. On the go, you can buy chlorophyll in drop form and add it to your drinks.

Green Juice

6–7 baby carrots
1 Granny Smith apple
3–4 stalks of celery
1 small cucumber
3 cups finely chopped kale
1 peeled lime
Sea salt to taste

Juice the veggies and fruit in a juicer, and top it off with some sea salt. If you have blood sugar concerns, blend with 1–2 tablespoons of coconut oil or 1 avocado. This is my all-time favorite juice.

9. Fermented foods: Fermented foods are filled with probiotics that support gut and detox pathways. The bacteria found in the fermented foods can be beneficial in balancing your intestinal flora and can help with symptoms of constipation, digestion, and anxiety. Fermented coconut yogurt, fermented coconut water, and fermented cabbage are a few of my favorites. If you buy fermented foods, including cabbage, be sure to pick the kind that are kept in the fridge. Probiotic bacteria can only survive a couple of weeks at room temperature.

10. Turmeric: Curcumin, the active ingredient in turmeric, is great for detoxifying various metals and toxins. Turmeric has a great taste and, added to hot water, is an excellent choice to replace hot tea. Turmeric powder has anti-inflammatory, detoxifying, antioxidant, antibacterial, and antiviral properties. Typically, the effects of curcumin only last about an hour in the body, but I've found that combining curcumin with piperine, an alkaloid found in pepper, will keep it in the body longer.

A simple way to incorporate turmeric is to add it to your cooking (remember to add some pepper to the mix as well). After my arsenic poisoning, I used curcumin to detoxify my body, and I believe that the addition of turmeric helped me eliminate the arsenic within a month and prevent long-term damage.

I recommend turmeric for clients with Hashimoto's to support the liver and inflammatory pathways. You can enjoy turmeric tea twice per day and eat tandoori chicken multiple times per week.

Turmeric Tea

1 teaspoon turmeric
1 teaspoon ginger
Pinch of pepper
Pinch of cinnamon
Juice of 1 lemon
Sweetener to taste (stevia and maple syrup are my top recommendations)
1 cup hot filtered water

Put all the spices and lemon juice in the mug of your choice, top off with boiling water, and mix!

Tandoori Chicken

1 teaspoon curry

1 teaspoon turmeric

1 teaspoon paprika (skip if you are nightshade sensitive)

1 teaspoon garlic powder

½ teaspoon pepper

1 teaspoon sea salt

2 cups coconut milk

1 whole chicken, cut up, or 8 chicken drumsticks

Add all ingredients to slow cooker and cook on medium for 8 hours.

11. Berries: Berries are full of phytonutrients and antioxidants, and they are less likely to spike your blood sugar compared to other fruit. Furthermore, blueberries are a rich source of myo-inositol, a nutrient that has been shown to improve thyroid function and blood sugar. Many people already love blackberries, blueberries, raspberries, and strawberries, and you may also find that some exotic berries like boysenberries, currants, and gooseberries are delicious as well. If you can, try to buy organic fruit with limited exposure to pesticides.

I generally recommend aiming for ½ to 1 cup of berries a day, depending on your blood sugar levels, and eating them toward the evening. If you ingest too much fruit in the morning, this can cause spikes in your blood sugar, leaving you tired throughout the day. It's important to practice moderation, even with fruit, as too much fructose has been linked to insulin resistance and fatty liver disease.

Transitioning to a Nutrient-Dense Plan

As you work to include more of these nutrient-dense foods, I also want to caution you against gravitating toward certain gluten-free processed foods. I know when I first changed my diet, I ended up on a GFJF diet—a gluten-free junk food diet! This is when you replace your gluten-filled junk foods with gluten-free junk foods. While this is a step up from eating gluten, GFJF is still junk food and won't get you very far on your healing journey.

If you must, I recommend consuming GFJF items like gluten-free pancake mixes, cookies, cereals, and breads only in the transition process if you have been eating the standard American diet. Most gluten-free foods will still spike up your blood sugar (taxing your adrenals, which can weaken the thyroid), and may contain thyroid-harmful ingredients like soy. We will dive deeper into optimizing your nutrition in later chapters.

So, What's for Breakfast?

You might have noticed that these exclusions eliminate a lot of your favorite breakfast items—no more cereal, waffles, or toast. But don't worry: I have some new breakfast ideas for you. Here are some of my favorites:

The SGC

Smoked wild-caught salmon
Guacamole (avocado, garlic powder, tomatoes,* onions)
Fermented cabbage

Add all ingredients to a plate and enjoy!

*Avoid if you have a nightshade sensitivity.

Breakfast Hash

1 pound grass-fed ground beef

4 cups chopped mixture of zucchini, carrots, broccoli, cauliflower

¼ cup chopped onion

Stir-fry 10–15 minutes until veggies and meat are cooked through. Tip: Make a big batch and freeze in breakfast-size portions.

Root Cause Smoothie

12 ounces coconut milk

1 scoop pea protein/hemp protein/beef protein, as tolerated

2 cups chopped mixture of lettuce, celery, carrots

Lemon juice/lime juice to taste

1 avocado

Juice all ingredients in a blender and enjoy.

Breakfast Spaghetti

1 medium squash (spaghetti, acorn, or butternut)

1 cup cooked diced chicken, beef, or pork

1 tablespoon coconut oil

1 teaspoon basil

Sea salt to taste

Water

Before bed, put the squash in a slow cooker. Add the diced meat, coconut oil, basil, and sea salt. Cover with water. Cook on low overnight. Wake up to great smells in the morning!

Breakfast Delight

Coconut oil

1 cup diced butternut squash

1 pound chicken tenders

1 cup baby kale

1 teaspoon basil

Sea salt to taste

Olive oil to taste

Stir-fry in coconut oil for 10 minutes. Top with olive oil to serve.

Liver Support Recipes

Hot Lemon Water

Juice of 1 lemon

1 cup hot filtered water

Stevia to taste

Add lemon juice to hot water and sweeten to taste. Drink first thing in the morning instead of caffeine.

Detox Juice

1 bunch cilantro

1 cup coconut water

Stevia to taste

Juice of ½ lemon

10 drops chlorophyll

Hot filtered water

Blend all ingredients and enjoy.

Peppermint Tea

1 bunch of peppermint
1 cup hot filtered water
Stevia to taste

Add peppermint to the hot water and let steep for five minutes. Remove mint, sweeten to taste, and enjoy!

Spa Water

1 pitcher filtered water
¼ cup each of mint, halved strawberries, and cut cucumbers

Add mint, strawberries, and cucumber to water. Sip throughout the day.

Maca Latte

1 tablespoon maca powder
1 tablespoon coconut milk
1 teaspoon cinnamon
Stevia to taste
1 cup hot filtered water

Add all ingredients to a blender and blend until smooth. Enjoy!

Fermented Margarita

1 cup fermented coconut water
Juice of 1 lime
½ teaspoon sea salt
Stevia to taste

Mix ingredients in a glass. Add ice and blend if desired. Trust me, it's yummy!

Virgin Mojito

Juice of 1 lime
1 bunch mint leaves
½ teaspoon ground ginger
1 cup filtered water or coconut water
Stevia to taste

Mash mint leaves using a mortar and pestle to release the flavor. Mix with the rest of the ingredients in a glass, and enjoy. Alternatively, place all ingredients into a blender and blend.

Combining the First Two Steps: The Easy Liver Support Food Plan

Now that you have an understanding of what trigger foods to avoid and what superfoods to add, I want to share with you a simple overview of how your diet might look over the next two weeks. Eating a clean, nutrient-dense diet doesn't have to be complicated!

Breakfasts and Snacks

Breakfast and snacks will consist of green smoothies. You can make the Root Cause Green Smoothie (see page 119) or create your own. Just be sure to include these three components:

- **Fiber:** The green smoothies should include a mix of vegetables, including green leafy vegetables, and a small serving of berries for antioxidants or a banana.
- **Fat:** Coconut milk and avocados can be used for a yummy source of good fat.

- **Protein:** A hypoallergenic protein like pea protein or hydrolyzed beef protein is my top recommendation.

SAMPLE DAILY MEAL PLAN

Time	Food/Drink
7:00 A.M.	Hot Lemon Water
8:00 A.M.	Root Cause Green Smoothie
10:00 A.M.	Green Juice
12:00 P.M.	Salad
3:00 P.M.	Peppermint Tea or Maca Latte
6:00 P.M.	Dinner with organic meats and veggies
8:00 P.M.	Detox Juice, Fermented Margarita, or Virgin Mojito

A simple hack for people who work (or have a life) is to precut all of the veggies you'll need for the week and put them in thirty-two-ounce, wide-mouth Mason jars on Sunday night. Each morning, throw the veggies and fruit, coconut milk or avocado, and powdered protein into the blender, adding water to desired consistency. Enjoy before you head out the door to start your day.

Lunches

Keep it simple by having your lunches consist of salads with plenty of good fats, fiber, and protein.

- **Fats:** Use olive oil, olives, avocados, nuts, seeds, and coconut shavings.
- **Fiber:** Use chopped carrots, tomatoes, chopped cucumbers, lettuces, berries, and artichokes.
- **Protein:** Use cooked chicken, boiled egg, steak, shredded meat, meatballs, nuts, and seeds.

You can top it off with a healthy dressing. I recommend mixing extra virgin olive oil, lemon juice, and herbs like basil or oregano together.

You can simplify your lunch with Mason jars as well. I use five sixteen- or thirty-two-ounce jars and fill each with a mixture of chopped vegetables for each day of week. Stack your hard vegetables (like cut cucumber, bell peppers, and baby carrots) at the bottom of the jar, followed by softer veggies and fruit (like cherry tomatoes or blueberries). Layer with olives, nuts, seeds, and coconut shavings. You can even add olive oil, lemon, and herbs to the top. Keep avocados and proteins in a separate container. When you're ready to eat, mix the veggies and fruits with the proteins and dressing on a plate or in a big container.

Dinners

Keeping the same balance in mind for dinner, focus on generous servings of organic meats and veggies. Be sure to include crucifers like broccoli, cauliflower, Brussels sprouts, kale, cabbage, and turnips. Organic vegetables are best.

Batch cooking and slow cooking are some of my favorite simplifications for keeping dinnertime low maintenance.

Step 3: Reduce Toxic Exposure

While we like to think of our homes as our sanctuaries, they also have countless places for toxins to hide, including in the kitchen, bedroom, and bathroom. Removing small daily exposures in your home life can make a big difference in your symptoms in as little as two weeks, especially when combined with the other strategies in this chapter.

Following are some practical tips that will help you greatly reduce your daily toxic burden.

Green Your Kitchen

There are many places in the kitchen for toxic substances to hide. They can be lurking in cookware, food storage containers, utensils, and more. Here are some steps you can take to minimize toxins in the kitchen:

- Ditch your Teflon, stainless steel, and plastic cooking utensils for less toxic options for cooking: glass baking dishes, ceramic-coated pots and pans, and cast-iron skillets. Cast-iron skillets offer an extra bonus for people who struggle with anemia and low ferritin levels—these skillets will help you get your daily dose of iron.
- Use wood utensils to cook, stir, and stir-fry instead of plastic-coated or metal utensils.
- Chlorine-free parchment paper can be a suitable replacement for aluminum foil in baking, grilling, and steaming.
- Replace your plastic food storage containers with glass containers. My favorites are wide-mouthed glass Mason jars. If you use plastic at all, look for BPA-free plastic products. This includes storage bags, such as Ziploc brand, which are BPA-free. The best option is to avoid cooking or storing your food in plastics.
- Avoid the use of antibacterial products. They are not necessary in most homes. If you must use an antimicrobial product for work or disinfecting purposes, choose an alcohol hand rub or rinse product that does not list triclosan or any fragrance in the ingredients.

Green Your Water

Removing chemicals such as fluoride and chlorine from your water is an important step in reducing your toxic exposure. Since these and other chemicals are found in our public water supplies, you'll have to use a reverse osmosis filter to remove them. If you do not have a filter or if you live in an apartment, you may want to drink bottled water or get a fluoride-free water delivery service to come to your home.

Bottled water brands that contain less than <0.1 ppm of fluoride include Aquafina, Calistoga, and Dasani. Please be sure to periodically check www.fluoridealert.org/content/bottled-water/, as companies may change their practices without warning. Drinking from plastic bottles is not ideal due to the potential toxicity of the plastic—thus, in the long run, I do recommend investing in a fluoride filter.

For brands of reverse osmosis filters, please go to www.thyroidphar macist.com/action.

Green Your Air

I recommend getting an air purifier for your home (especially your bedroom) to clear out airborne toxins. A less industrial and more decorative option includes getting the type of houseplants that act as natural air detoxifiers. Golden Pothos, corn plants, and any of the *Sansevieria* genus have been used as purifiers and have gained a reputation for even being able to mitigate the effects of sick building syndrome. *Sansevieria* absorb carbon dioxide and release oxygen at night, making them excellent bedroom plants. However, as their leaves are poisonous if ingested, they should be kept out of reach of children and pets. Pet lovers, be aware that all of these plants can be poisonous to cats and dogs if ingested by the critters, so remember to keep them away from your fur babies.

Detox Personal Care

During the two-week Liver Support Protocol, I recommend that you go on a beauty detox to minimize your use of conventional personal care items such as shampoos, lotions, makeup, antiperspirants, and perfumes. Yes, ladies, all of the magic potions and lotions and lipsticks you use each day!

If you could go without makeup for two weeks, that would be best. However, if you are not too excited about the prospect of going makeup-free, look for clean brands at your local health food store. It's difficult to recommend makeup brands, as I know everyone has different complexions and needs, but here are some brands I have found to be both low in toxins and effective:

- **Makeup:** bareMinerals and Physicians Formula Organic Wear
- **Shampoo:** Acure Organics
- **Body wash:** Acure Organics, Dr. Bronner's

- **Lotion:** Acure Organics
- **Skin care:** MyChelle, Annmarie Gianni Skin Care, The Spa Dr.

For perfume, try mixing a blend of essential oils you like. I really enjoy the smell of frankincense, rose, and lavender together, though everyone has their personal preference. If you are not an oil connoisseur, you can purchase premade essential-oil-based perfumes like the Aura Cacia chakra roll-ons. The Expressive Throat aromatherapy roll-on smells like my high-end department store perfumes without the added toxins!

While I haven't tested this personally, some of my friends and colleagues, like nutritionist Carrie Vitt from Deliciously Organic, swear by using essential oils like frankincense, clove, myrrh, marjoram, basil, and lemongrass to support thyroid function naturally. (You can find links to all of my favorite products on my website www .thyroidpharmacist.com/action.)

If you need some added encouragement for greening your makeup and personal care routine, check out the website www.safecosmetics .org or search www.ewg.org/skindeep/search to see how your current products rate.

Step 4: Support Detox Pathways

Avoiding alcohol, caffeine, pesticides, and chemicals is a great way to kick-start the detoxification process. However, sometimes additional interventions may be required to help the body process a toxic backlog. Here are some activities and supplements you can add to the protocol to further boost detoxification.

Sweating

Sweating is an excellent way to lower your body's toxic burden. As people with hypothyroidism usually have a lower body temperature, they often need to make an extra effort to sweat. This can be done by exercise, the use of saunas, hot baths, or my favorite: hot yoga.

Sweating induced by hot springs, hot saunas, hot baths, hot yoga, or other forms of exercise can help us get rid of toxins at a quicker rate. Just don't overdo it, and please use good judgment. As a general rule, you should feel more energized after these activities, not more tired.

My clients with Hashimoto's often tell me they feel much better after a session in an infrared sauna or a hot yoga session. A DIY option in your own home may consist of taking a hot Epsom salt bath with some essential oils added to the tub.

Liver Support Supplements

Clients have reported that adding liver support supplements can accelerate the results they get from the Liver Support Protocol and dramatically improve how they feel. The liver utilizes two main chemical pathways for detox, and if either pathway is blocked, you won't be able to get rid of toxins. If we only support one path, a buildup of intermediates will cause more harm than good. Luckily, we can add supplements that may help open up both of these important detox pathways.

The Phase 1 Pathway utilizes chemical processes like oxidation, reduction, hydrolysis, hydration, and dehalogenation of fat-soluble toxins. Toxins live inside our fat cells, and we need nutrients like B_2, B_3, B_5, B_6, B_{12}, folate, glutathione, and flavonoids to get them out and turn them into intermediates that can be eliminated in Phase 2 correctly. An important thing to note is that after toxins go through Phase 1, the intermediate products may actually be more toxic! This is when Phase 2 kicks in.

The Phase 2 Pathway is the second step of the process, and the essential role of this pathway is to help eliminate the waste created in Phase 1. This process includes sulfation, glucuronidation, glutathione conjugation, acetylation, amino acid conjugation, and methylation. *Methylation will be impaired if you have the MTHFR gene mutation.* Phase 2 needs nutrients like methionine, cysteine, magnesium, glutathione, vitamins B_5 and B_{12}, vitamin C, glycine, taurine, glutamine, folate, and choline. Methylsulfonylmethane

(MSM) and N-acetylcysteine (NAC) are also two helpful supplements to help this pathway along.

The list of required nutrients for Phases 1 and 2 liver detoxification include B vitamins (B_2, B_3, B_5, B_6, B_{12}), folate, glutathione, flavonoids, magnesium, vitamin C, and the amino acids methionine, cysteine, glycine, taurine, and glutamine.

To simplify things, I like utilizing products that have ingredients that support both liver detoxification pathways at once and have had great results with specialized pea protein powders that add in liver support nutrients.

Another important substance that aids the liver with clearing toxins is bile. Bile is a liquid that is produced by the liver and concentrated in the gallbladder. Bile has the important role of helping us with breaking down fats from foods for digestion and fats from toxins for elimination.

Poor bile flow has been associated with hypothyroidism and may lead to a recirculation of toxins as well as fat malabsorption; deficiencies in fatty acids and the vitamins A, D, E, and K; and retention of toxins.

Impairments in bile flow can also be caused by removal of the gallbladder, pancreatic deficiency, a congested liver, SIBO, and gallstones.

L-methionine, taurine, inositol, choline, milk thistle, dandelion, artichoke, beets, beta-carotene, and ox bile supplements can help support the liver and bile flow to ensure proper absorption of essential fats and vitamins as well as elimination of toxins. Gallbladder-supporting supplements usually contain a mixture of the above ingredients.

I'll highlight some of the important liver support supplements that you may want to take over this two-week protocol. Also, on pages 143–144, you'll find a chart that includes supplements, doses, and recommended brands.

NAC

Glutathione deficiency has been implicated with a higher level of thyroid antibodies. NAC, which turns into glutathione, not only helps

Root Cause Research Corner: Toxins in Supplements

I recommend exercising extreme caution with the use of supplements. A study done by JAMA in August of 2008 found that 20 percent of Ayurvedic medicines sold via the internet contained lead, mercury, and arsenic. Since 1978, more than eighty cases of lead poisoning have been associated with Ayurvedic medicine.

Ayurvedic medicines come in two major types: herbal only and *rasa shastra*. Rasa shastra is an ancient practice of mixing herbs with metals, minerals, and gems, including mercury, lead, iron, zinc, mica, and pearl. Rasa shastra formulations are twice as likely to contain heavy metals. In the study, several formulations had lead and mercury amounts of 100 to 10,000 times of allowable amounts! These preparations can be especially problematic for people with over-burdened detox pathways like those with Hashimoto's and MTHFR gene mutation.

I trust only high-quality professional supplement brands (see page 143) and have gone a step further and formulated my own line of supplements, which undergoes extensive testing for heavy metals, toxins, and contamination.

reduce thyroid antibodies by neutralizing hydrogen peroxide, but it also helps heal intestinal permeability and aids with detoxification. Doses of 1.8 g (1,800 mg) are usually recommended.

Amino Acids

Amino acids are necessary for detoxifying and rebuilding the body. Proteins are our major source of amino acids. However, protein breakdown is a burdensome process for the body and may be incomplete in those with Hashimoto's. Rather than increasing protein intake past appropriate weight and activity levels, taking pure amino acids may be a more viable option. (To learn how to calculate your protein requirements, please see page 179). Pure amino acids require no work on the part of the body and are easily absorbable. Pure amino acids may be taken in powder or supplement form.

Supplements that contain amino acids and support liver detox (glutamine, glycine, taurine, alpha-ketoglutarate, glutathione, methionine, ornithine) are especially important.

Curcumin

We already talked about the benefits of adding curcumin (in the form of turmeric) to your foods and beverages. While this will be beneficial—and delicious—curcumin in this form can be quickly excreted out of the body. In supplement form, curcumin should be in a suspended release formulation or combined with piperine, an alkaloid found in pepper, to remain active for a longer time in the body.

Herbs

I have found a variety of herbs to be helpful with cleansing, including MSM, dandelion, quercetin, and milk thistle. The antioxidant quercetin, specifically, can mitigate the toxicity of BPA in the body. Herbs can be purchased individually, but it's often more practical to use liver support powdered supplement blends that combine herbs with liver-supporting vitamins and minerals.

Methylation-Support Supplements

You can support methylation pathways by taking supplements with activated B_6 (as pyridoxal-5-phosphate), activated folate, and B_{12} as methylcobalamin and trimethylglycine, which breaks down homocysteine. For most people with Hashimoto's, I recommend this support for at least for two weeks during the protocol. Those with the MTHFR gene mutation will likely benefit from long-term supplementation.

Genetic Variations in Detox Capabilities

Some individuals with Hashimoto's may have a variation in the MTHFR gene that prevents them from properly activating folate, an important substance needed for detoxification pathways. This gene variation is present in up to 55 percent of the European population, and some have been saying that this variation seems to be more common in those with autoimmune disease.

The MTHFR gene codes for the MTHFR enzyme, the enzyme that converts the amino acid homocysteine to methionine, which is needed to make proteins in the body. Individuals with low activity of the MTHFR enzyme may present with elevated homocysteine levels, which have been associated with inflammation, blood clots, heart disease, birth defects, difficult pregnancies, and potentially an impaired ability to detoxify.

Nutrient deficiencies in folate, B_6, and B_{12} have also been associated with elevated homocysteine. However, individuals with the MTHFR gene actually have a difficult time processing the folic acid, B_6, and B_{12} that is present in most cheap supplements and added to processed foods. Some professionals claim that this synthetic folic acid may even cause a buildup in the body, leading to toxicity and an increased cancer risk—one more reason to ditch processed foods and cheap multivitamins!

Given the frequency and significance of the MTHFR gene mutation, I recommend methylated versions of B_6, B_{12}, and folate combined with other homocysteine-reducing interventions for most of my clients with Hashimoto's. Individuals without the gene defect will benefit from the short-term support utilized in the Liver Support Protocol of this book (two weeks), while those with the gene mutation will benefit from long-term support. You can read more about the MTHFR support nutrients in this chapter, and we will cover the MTHFR gene in more detail in chapter 12.

Magnesium

Magnesium is a powerhouse nutrient when it comes to detoxification. Magnesium is required for the liver's detoxification pathways, for alkalizing the body so that toxins can leave through the urine more readily, and for helping to rid the body of toxins with more frequent bowel movements.

Magnesium deficiency is very common in the general population and may affect as many as 70 percent of people. Deficiency has been tied to trouble falling asleep, muscle twitching and cramps, premenstrual syndrome, restless leg syndrome, palpitations, poor mood, irritability, anxiety, headaches and migraines, acid reflux, sensitivity to loud noises, and constipation.

Many of my clients have found that taking a bedtime magnesium supplement helped them fall and stay asleep, reduced headaches, reduced muscle pains and cramps, eliminated menstrual cramps, and lessened feelings of anxiety. This anecdotal evidence matches up with the research, which has shown that when people with autoimmune thyroid disease took magnesium citrate for six weeks, they reported feeling better with more energy, better sleep, less anxiety, and less constipation. These patients also had reductions in TSH, dropping from an average of 7.67 µIU/mL to 2.67 µIU/mL! One person's TSH even dropped by 17 points, from 21 µIU/mL to 4 µIU/mL.

The researchers who conducted this study, Roy and Helga Moncayo of Austria, who've been studying Hashimoto's for nearly ten years, also reported a normalization of damage on some of the patients' thyroid ultrasounds after eight months of supplementation with magnesium.

Magnesium citrate and magnesium glycinate are great sources of oral magnesium supplements. Magnesium citrate has more stool-softening properties and also tends to be more calming than the glycinate, so this is something to consider based on your bowel function and may be more appropriate for people with anxiety. Usual starting dose ranges for magnesium are: magnesium citrate at 400 mg or magnesium glycinate at 100 mg at bedtime. Be sure to give yourself four hours between your thyroid medications and your magnesium dose. If you experience diarrhea, this could be an indication that you are getting too much magnesium and that you should lower your dose or perhaps switch to a different version.

Best High-Quality Supplement Brands

As a pharmacist I am well aware that all supplements are not created equally. Vitamin and supplement companies do not undergo the same scrutiny as do pharmaceutical products. This can result in ineffective and even dangerous products.

Here's what you should look for when choosing supplements:

- Supplements should be free of artificial additives, gluten, and dairy. Even small amounts can be detrimental and interfere with absorption.
- Methylated forms of B_{12} (methylcobalamin) are more bioavailable than cyanocobalamin versions.
- Folic acid should be in the form of methylfolate, Metafolin, or NatureFolate, especially for those with MTHFR gene variations.
- Formulations should be tested for purity, and the supplements should be tested to make sure the contents match the label description.

I have spent a great deal of time researching and testing various supplement brands, but I've always been hesitant to recommend specific brands or even products that I created. I didn't want people to think that I was giving them biased information because of my relationship with a specific company or, worse, that I was only sharing information to sell my own products!

This is why in my first book I kept recommendations to a minimum. However, numerous clients and readers have asked for specific

Liver Support Supplements

Supplement	How to Use	Recommended Brands
MTHFR support supplement with activated B_6 (as pyridoxal-5-phosphate), activated folate, B_{12} as methylcobalamin and trimethylglycine	Take daily during detox, and continue indefinitely if you have the MTHFR gene mutation.	Rootcology Methylation Support, Pure Encapsulations Homocysteine Factors, Designs for Health Homocysteine Supreme
Supplement containing amino acids to support phase 2 liver detox (glutamine, glycine, taurine, alpha-ketoglutarate, glutathione, methionine, ornithine)	Take 6 capsules daily during 2-week liver protocol and continue during gut cleanse.	Rootcology Amino Support, Designs for Health Amino-D-Tox
Supplement containing gallbladder, liver, and bile flow supporting substances (L-methionine, taurine, inositol, choline, beta-carotene, ox bile, milk thistle, dandelion, artichoke, beet)	Take 3 capsules daily during 2-week liver protocol. May continue beyond if experiencing fat malabsorption/gallbladder issues.	Rootcology Liver Gallbladder Support, Pure Encapsulations Digestion GB, LV-GB by Designs for Health
NAC	Take 1,800 mg daily with food, starting with liver support, and continue for 3–6 months.	Rootcology, Pure Encapsulations, Designs for Health
Curcumin with bioperine	Take 1–3 capsules daily during 2-week liver support.	Pure Encapsulations

Supplement	How to Use	Recommended Brands
Liver support powder containing amino acids, nutrients, and herbs	Add 1 scoop to smoothies for 2 weeks.	Rootcology Liver Reset Powder, Designs for Health PaleoCleanse
Magnesium (citrate or glycinate)	Take 1–4 capsules at bedtime starting with liver support and may continue for 3–6 months or as needed.	Pure Encapsulations

recommendations and brands, and many have even asked that I formulate my own line of products. This type of feedback inspired me to create Rootcology, my own line of supplements, as I wanted to be sure that my clients were getting consistent results with my recommendations.

Additionally, some of my favorite high-quality brands include Pure Encapsulations, Designs for Health, Douglas Laboratories, Bulletproof, NOW Foods, Protocol for Life Balance, Metagenics, Vital Nutrients, Thorne, and Allergy Research Group.

Please note that at times formulations may change. This is another reason I created Rootcology—I now have control of all of the ingredients, additives, and test procedures, thus I can feel comfortable recommending them. You can be sure that you are getting a high-quality, safe, and effective supplement.

The Liver Support Supplements table is a summary of all the recommended supplements that will assist in your healing during the Liver Support Protocol.

How You'll Feel with the Supplements

Most people report feeling more energetic, while some report feeling more tired on the recommended liver support supplements. While sensitivity reactions are possible to any ingredient in any product, to date, the only adverse reactions reported by my clients who were using my recommended liver support supplements were those due to easily corrected magnesium deficiency, such as constipation, headaches, muscle tightness, or insomnia. This is because magnesium becomes depleted as toxins begin to leave the body. Therefore, please note that magnesium requirements may increase while taking liver support supplements.

Additional Interventions and Protocols

Once you've completed the two-week protocol, be sure to retake the Liver Assessment from pages 84–85. What changes and improvements did you notice?

While many people will be able to flush a toxic buildup by following the steps outlined in the Liver Support Protocol, some individuals with a significant heavy metal burden may require further interventions. I recommend completing the Adrenal Recovery and Gut Balance Protocols and then retesting your toxicity score. If your toxicity score is still elevated after you've completed all three Fundamental Protocols, be sure to reference the Advanced Protocols in chapter 12.

Now, it's time to move on to your adrenals! If you feel noticeably better after the Liver Support Protocol but can't shake low energy, feelings of agitation, brain fog, or general malaise, you likely have underlying adrenal dysfunction. Restoring your adrenal glands to proper working order is the essential next step in your recovery.

5

Adrenal Recovery Protocol

Those of us with Hashimoto's often blame our thyroid for the many symptoms we experience. Hair loss? Thyroid! Weight gain? Thyroid! Fatigue? It's gotta be the thyroid! But my experience both in working with Hashimoto's patients and in treating my own condition has revealed that there is typically another player involved in hypothyroidism: the adrenals, or to be more exact, the hormones produced by the adrenal glands. In fact, I've found that 90 percent of Hashimoto's patients are dealing with at least some degree of adrenal dysfunction. (Please note, this condition is more accurately referred to as hypothalamic-pituitary axis dysfunction, adrenal insufficiency, or hypocortisolism, but to keep with common language of use, I will refer to it as adrenal dysfunction.)

Dysfunction in adrenal hormone production is often to blame for symptoms that don't seem to retreat even after thyroid hormone treatment is in progress. After starting thyroid hormones, a person with adrenal dysfunction might initially report feeling more energetic but then find that she gradually starts to feel worse until she's right back to where she was before beginning thyroid treatment. A trip back to her physician to check blood work will likely suggest that her thyroid function is normal.

But most blood tests will not reveal adrenal dysfunction. And most conventional medicine doctors won't run any additional or proper tests for it, such as adrenal saliva or urinary stress hormone panels, because they do not consider adrenal dysfunction as a real condition.

This is unfortunate because most people with Hashimoto's are likely to have numerous signs and symptoms of adrenal dysfunction, which may be worsening thyroid symptoms and could potentially have even been the trigger for their thyroid disease. The adrenals and thyroid gland have an intricate feedback loop, and taking thyroid medications without adrenal support can negatively impact adrenal function and thus symptoms in the long term. Therefore, supporting adrenal hormones is a really important part of overcoming Hashimoto's.

Adrenal hormone imbalance may initiate or exacerbate the following symptoms: feeling overwhelmed, feeling tired despite adequate sleep, difficulty getting up in the morning, craving salty foods (aka "I just ate a whole bag of chips" syndrome), increased effort required for everyday activities, low blood pressure, feeling faint when getting up quickly, mental fog, alternating diarrhea and constipation, low blood sugar, decreased sex drive, decreased ability to handle stress, slowed healing, mild depression, less enjoyment in life, feeling worse after skipping meals, increased PMS, poor concentration, reduced ability to make decisions, reduced productivity, and poor memory. Do any of these sound familiar? The adrenal assessment will help determine your risk for impaired adrenal function.

ADRENAL ASSESSMENT

Mark the symptoms that apply to you currently.

☐ I have low blood pressure.
☐ I feel dizzy when I stand up.
☐ I have hypoglycemia (low blood sugar).
☐ I crave salt.
☐ I crave sweets.
☐ I have dark circles under my eyes.
☐ I have sleep problems (either falling asleep or staying asleep).
☐ I have nonrestorative sleep (don't feel reenergized).

☐ I have mental fogginess or trouble concentrating.
☐ I have headaches.
☐ I have frequent infections (catch cold easily).
☐ I don't tolerate exercise well and feel completely exhausted after.
☐ I feel stressed most of the time.
☐ I feel tired but wired.
☐ I retain water.
☐ I have panic attacks or am easily startled.
☐ I have heart palpitations.
☐ I need to start the day with caffeine.
☐ I have poor tolerance to alcohol, caffeine, and other drugs.
☐ I feel weak and shaky.
☐ I have sweaty palms and feet when nervous.
☐ I feel fatigued.
☐ I felt worse shortly after taking thyroid medications.
☐ Fasting makes me feel worse.
☐ My muscles are weak.

Total number of symptoms: ___

<3: Low risk
3–6: Intermediate risk
>7: High risk

This chapter will give you the fundamental recommendations to support your adrenals, especially optimizing sleep, correcting blood sugar imbalances, minimizing stress, and reducing inflammation through food modifications. If you've already cut out gluten, dairy, and soy, you're off to a great start. This chapter will cover additional reactive foods, and the rest of the book will progressively guide you to reduce the inflammation in your body.

The complete five-step Adrenal Recovery Protocol will look like this:

1. Rest.
2. De-stress.
3. Reduce inflammation.

4. Balance the blood sugar.

5. Replenish nutrients and add adaptogens.

Before we dive into the interventions, let's talk about the adrenal glands and how functional problems can develop here.

Getting to Know the Adrenal Glands

The adrenal glands are organs that sit on top of each kidney. They are known as our stress glands because they produce a variety of hormones necessary for our survival. Each gland has two separate zones: the inner zone, or medulla, secretes the hormones epinephrine (also known as adrenaline), norepinephrine, and a small amount of dopamine in response to immediate stress signaled by the central nervous system.

The outer zone of the adrenal gland is known as the cortex. The cortex secretes three types of hormones: glucocorticoids, mineralocorticoids, and androgens. These hormones are made from cholesterol and secreted in varied amounts throughout the day in a rhythmic pattern, with the highest amounts in the morning and the lowest at night. When the adrenal glands are not putting out sufficient amounts of hormones or the rhythm becomes disturbed, adrenal dysfunction develops.

The most important adrenal hormone is cortisol. Cortisol has several important jobs, including helping regulate our blood sugar and body fat, protecting the body against infections, and helping us to adapt to stress. Cortisol also manages inflammation and is involved in the process that converts food into energy.

These are the other important adrenal hormones:

• **Pregnenolone:** Pregnenolone is the first hormone made from cholesterol and is the precursor, or mother hormone, for DHEA, estrogen, testosterone, progesterone, aldosterone, and cortisol. This means that levels of these important hormones depend on the availability of pregnenolone. Pregnenolone may help boost your resistance to stress and play an important role in memory function.

- **Aldosterone:** The main mineralocorticoid, aldosterone helps to regulate blood volume, blood pressure, and the body's sodium and potassium levels.
- **Dehydroepiandrosterone:** DHEA has been touted as the youth hormone due to peak production taking place at age twenty then declining with age. DHEA helps us manage growth hormone, which is a powerful antiaging hormone, and also helps us make sufficient amounts of the sex hormones estrogen and testosterone. Deficiencies in DHEA have been implicated in low libido, and a 2014 study found that women with Hashimoto's and premature ovarian failure were more likely to have low levels of DHEA. DHEA supplementation has also shown to help reduce thyroid antibodies.

As adrenal hormones are precursors of sex hormones and contribute to the overall hormonal load, it's easy to see how adrenal hormones can often be the root cause of other hormonal imbalances and symptoms like premenstrual syndrome, low libido, irregular menses, and even infertility. So what causes the adrenals to become imbalanced? Let's take a look at how the process unravels—it actually involves not just the adrenal glands but the hypothalamus and the pituitary gland too.

How the HPA Axis and Too Much Stress Collide to Create Adrenal Fatigue

In most cases of adrenal fatigue, the problems originate in a communication breakdown that occurs within the hypothalamic-pituitary-adrenal axis, otherwise known as the HPA axis. The HPA axis describes the interactive feedback loop that takes place between these three endocrine glands.

The hypothalamus is like the CEO of our body's production of hormones. It scans messages from our environment and other endocrine glands and checks the body's overall hormonal status before passing on the order for more hormones to the pituitary gland. The pituitary gland then acts as a project manager and pulls together individual workers (like the thyroid gland, the adrenal gland, and the gonads) to do their jobs. The pituitary will also make sure the workers have adequate resources to do their jobs by managing growth (and repair) and electrolyte-water balance. The HPA axis also controls milk production, such as in breastfeeding or galactorrhea, a hormonal imbalance of inappropriate milk secretion from the breasts. HPA axis dysfunction is one potential reason why some women with Hashimoto's may have poor milk production for breastfeeding on one end of the spectrum or unwanted milk production outside of pregnancy or breastfeeding (often associated with elevations of the hormone prolactin) on the other end of the spectrum.

The HPA axis works in response to two types of stress: immediate stress and chronic stress. Let's see how the responses to each type differ.

In cases of immediate stress, the hypothalamus senses stress and sets off a hormone cascade that leads to the activation of your fight-or-flight response (via the sympathetic nervous system). As part of this response, the adrenals pump out extra hormones, and your body goes from the parasympathetic state of relaxing, digesting, and healing to a survival state. Your body's energy is shifted from activities not essential to survival—like growing beautiful hair, metabolizing nutrients into energy, making hormones, and digesting and repairing itself—to instead focusing its resources on meeting the increased stress-induced demand for cortisol and adrenaline.

Then, once you've escaped from the bear or gotten out of the way of the oncoming car, the demand for emergency levels of hormones settles down and the focus once again turns to parasympathetic response, focused on body maintenance and upkeep.

In cases of chronic stress, the never-ending presence of situations that are stressful yet not life threatening can lead to the constant activation of the stress response. For example, the stress response might be cued when you're running late, stuck in traffic, dealing with a crying baby, or all of the above, leading to a relentless demand for hormones, especially cortisol.

To help meet the demand for cortisol, your body will decrease the production of other hormones normally produced by the adrenals, such as progesterone, DHEA, and testosterone, as a protective mechanism. If this protective process continues for too long, it can lead to deficiencies in the other hormones that depend on pregnenolone for production.

You can see, too, how constant stress might strain the HPA axis. The intense and immediate demand for hormones puts the entire process on overdrive, leaving room for a communication breakdown to occur. The HPA axis becomes overwhelmed and desensitized to the usual feedback loop, and it stops sending messages to the adrenals to produce more hormones. This is sometimes known as HPA axis suppression. Going back to the company examples, it's like the CEO gets tired of the employees always complaining about being overworked and stops giving them available projects, leading to a slowing down of the company. The employees are capable of doing more work, but they're not getting the messages that there is any more work.

Eventually, you might run out of nutrients that are required for proper adrenal function or your pituitary gland will no longer respond to the messages to produce stress hormones. When this happens, you will have reached a state of adrenal fatigue.

Checking Your Adrenal Health

Chronic stress can lead to progressively worse stages of adrenal dysfunction. In the early stages, the adrenals secrete excessive levels of cortisol; in the later stages, they secrete less and less, leading to inadequate levels of the anti-inflammatory hormone in the body.

Additionally, the levels of DHEA, one of our anabolic (building-up) hormones, drop as the adrenal dysfunction progresses.

While the adrenal assessment shared at the beginning of the chapter will help you determine if you have adrenal dysfunction, further testing is required to determine your precise stage of adrenal fatigue. The Adrenal Recovery Protocol strategies in this chapter will be helpful for all stages of adrenal dysfunction. Should you continue to have adrenal symptoms after finishing the protocol, please read chapter 10 for information on testing and targeted boosts for your precise stage of adrenal dysfunction, as well as to identify and resolve the root causes that may require additional interventions to heal.

Symptoms Over Time

HPA axis malfunction and the corresponding adrenal fatigue can lead to various symptoms, which can occur as chronic stress continues and the dysfunction moves from beginning to advanced stages.

Here are some of the symptoms and conditions that can occur:

- Low blood pressure, which happens in the advanced stages of adrenal fatigue as aldosterone production becomes depleted and levels of sodium and water drop. You might feel faint upon standing as a result of low blood pressure.
- Noticeable dehydration and cravings for salty foods (hello, potato chips!), and possibly an increase in potassium levels. In this case, foods containing high amounts of potassium might make you feel worse. Drinking more fluids will only result in further dilution of the sodium and increased dehydration.
- Seasonal depression, post-traumatic stress disorder, hypothyroidism, asthma, and eczema, all of which have all been linked to HPA axis malfunction.
- Menstrual irregularities, infertility, uterine fibroids, fibrocystic breasts, and a shift in immune function, all as a result of low progesterone.

- Elevated levels of cholesterol due to the body compensating for the increased need for this hormone-building material.

- Inflammatory bowel disease, rheumatoid arthritis, chronic fatigue syndrome, and fibromyalgia, which are linked to abnormally low levels of DHEA and progesterone.

The Connection Between Hashimoto's and Adrenal Fatigue

The symptoms of adrenal insufficiency experienced in Hashimoto's may be due to nutrient depletion, stress, miscommunication of the adrenal and pituitary glands, hormonal downregulation, or in rare cases, an autoimmune attack on the adrenals. If an autoimmune attack is being waged on the adrenal glands, a person has Addison's disease. Currently, this is the only adrenal insufficiency disorder recognized by conventional medical doctors.

When my integrative doctor first suggested I get tested for adrenal fatigue, I looked up the term and found what seemed to be a reputable source that stated adrenal fatigue was a made-up disorder and did not exist. Being a skeptical pharmacist, I decided to put off testing my adrenals. I had just ventured into the world of alternative medicine and was afraid of people trying to take advantage of me and take my money, not realizing that they were simply trying to help.

Eventually, I got to a point when I was just so exhausted and irritable, despite taking thyroid medications and following a gluten-free diet. I started talking to Carter Black, RPh, my compounding pharmacist, about the symptoms I was experiencing, and he suggested I have my adrenals tested. Mr. Black had specialized in hormones for many years and told me that the interventions for adrenal fatigue did indeed work well for many of his patients.

I was ready to keep digging—this time with an open mind. Maybe it was because I'd heard it from a fellow pharmacist or maybe it was because he didn't have anything to sell me that I decided to try

Root Cause Research Corner: What Is Addison's Disease?

People with Hashimoto's and other autoimmune disorders are more likely to develop Addison's disease, the autoimmune condition that results in the destruction of the adrenal glands.

Addison's is not usually diagnosed until 90 percent of the adrenal glands have been destroyed by autoimmune damage. At that point, a person presents with a potentially life-threatening adrenal crisis with potential symptoms of lethargy, low blood pressure, confusion, electrolyte imbalances, hypothyroidism, vomiting, diarrhea, and even convulsions.

However, antibodies to the adrenals, 21-hydroxylase antibodies, may be present for decades before an adrenal crisis sets in.

I believe that some individuals with Hashimoto's who also have symptoms of adrenal fatigue may actually have subclinical Addison's. This means the adrenals could be in the process of being destroyed, but the hormonal changes are yet to be significant enough to be detectable on blood tests—or the body may still be compensating.

If you want your conventional doctor to screen you for Addison's, you need to ask for an ACTH test and blood cortisol levels. Additionally, to detect the earlier stage of Addison's, it can be helpful to request a 21-hydroxylase autoantibody test despite normal ACTH and blood cortisol levels.

it. Sure enough, after taking an adrenal saliva test, I had an advanced stage of adrenal dysfunction, and the recommended treatments for the adrenal fatigue helped me feel tremendously better.

I now recommend the BioHealth adrenal saliva test to all of my clients with Hashimoto's, and I have found that 90 percent of the clients who do the test have some degree of adrenal dysfunction. Clients will say that they finally have more energy, lose weight, feel stronger, feel calmer, don't have crying fits, and have balanced libido and hormones after utilizing protocols for adrenal dysfunction. So trust me, and call it what you will, adrenal fatigue does exist!

How We Turn On Our Stress Response

There are four types of stress that turn on our fight-or-flight response (solutions to address each of these will be introduced later in the chapter):

- Inadequate sleep
- Mental and emotional stress
- Blood sugar imbalances
- Chronic inflammation

Inadequate Sleep

Sleep deprivation is a huge stressor on the body and contributes to adrenal imbalances, which then initiate the development of autoimmunity. Sleep deprivation is also the quickest way to get yourself into adrenal fatigue—in fact, sleep deprivation is what scientists use to induce HPA axis dysfunction in laboratory animals! A 2006 study found that shift workers, who typically have disrupted sleep patterns, were found to be at greater risk for developing thyroid antibodies compared to daytime workers.

Other research has linked sleep apnea, an increasingly common cause of sleep deprivation, to Hashimoto's. Sleep apnea is a chronic health condition that has been associated with low-grade inflammation in the body and is characterized by pauses in breathing while one is sleeping. As these pauses in breathing and lack of oxygen wake people up intermittently throughout the night, the result is often unrefreshing, fragmented sleep despite sleeping longer than usual.

Root Cause Research Corner: Obstructive Sleep Apnea and Hashimoto's

While hypothyroidism *can* cause sleep apnea due to protein deposits in the upper airway, increased risk of obesity, and abnormal control of ventilation, researchers wanted to know if obstructive sleep apnea (OSA) itself could be a trigger in Hashimoto's. They studied the incidence of thyroid antibodies in people with and without sleep apnea. Their results, which appeared in a 2012 study in *Endocrine* journal, showed that 53.2 percent of people with OSA were positive for TPO antibodies, TG antibodies, or both and thus had some stage of Hashimoto's. These people still had normal TSH numbers, so they had not yet developed hypothyroidism, suggesting that OSA may be a *causative* factor for Hashimoto's.

The more severe the sleep apnea, the more likely the subjects were to have Hashimoto's. Furthermore, men were especially affected: 66 percent of men with sleep apnea had Hashimoto's antibodies. Interestingly, when comparing Hashimoto's patients with and without sleep apnea, high levels of thyroid antibodies—in the range of 1,000 IU/mL or higher—seemed to be more common in those with sleep apnea. So if your antibodies are in the super-high range, consider this as a root cause, and as a Hashimoto's patient, remember to consider obstructive sleep apnea as a possible trigger.

The following symptoms have been correlated with sleep apnea: snoring, difficulty in waking up, restless sleep, nasal speech, mouth breathing, attention deficit disorder (especially in children), fatigue, and nasal congestion. People who snore at night should be suspected to have sleep apnea until proven otherwise.

Studies have found that 25 to 35 percent of people with hypothyroidism also have sleep apnea and that sleep apnea is also a risk factor for Hashimoto's.

You can get tested for sleep apnea, although it's not always easy, as it requires having your breathing monitored overnight at a sleep lab. Treatment consists of dental devices that advance the lower jaw, like the mandibular advancement device (MAD), or a continuous positive airway pressure (CPAP) machine to maintain breathing. If you have a small or receding jaw, thought to be caused by generations of processed food, mandibular advancement devices may be especially helpful. I also recommend looking for deeper root causes like infections that could contribute to symptoms of sleep apnea.

I've found that sleep apnea can be a potential root cause for Hashimoto's and adrenal fatigue. Clients with Hashimoto's who have used dental devices or the CPAP machine for sleep apnea reported feeling less fatigued and more energetic, and were finally able to make progress in their healing.

Mental and Emotional Stress

The most important strategy for combating adrenal fatigue is stress reduction. While this strategy does not involve dieting, supplements, medications, or testing, it can be the hardest to implement. Many people say this is the hardest lifestyle change for them to incorporate. Some of us only have two settings: go and sleep. I, like many of my clients, did not know how to relax, smell the roses, turn off, or unwind.

There are two keys to stress reduction. The first is to identify the things in your life that make you feel better and to do more of them. The second is to identify the things that make you feel worse and to eliminate as many as possible from your life. It sounds so simple, doesn't it?

Of course, there may be certain activities or experiences that make you feel worse that cannot be eliminated. For those things that you can't change, you can attempt to change your perception of them—usually it's not the event itself that makes us stressed out but our perception of it. A big part of changing your perception has to do with truly getting to know yourself and then honoring yourself for who you are rather than feeling guilty about who you may or may not be. This may be a simple shift of perspective for you, or it may require some deeper strategies, which will be covered in chapter 10.

Blood Sugar Imbalances

People often ask me if there is one thing that people with Hashimoto's could do right away to feel better, and the answer is yes: balance your blood sugar! Balancing blood sugar levels should be one of the priorities for anyone who is hoping to overcome autoimmune thyroiditis and adrenal fatigue. Reactive hypoglycemia, which is post-meal hypoglycemia that occurs within four hours of eating a high-carbohydrate meal, is in particular a huge stressor for the adrenals.

Blood sugar imbalances have been described as adding fuel to the fire in autoimmune thyroid disease by many practitioners who focus on reversing Hashimoto's.

Researchers in Poland have found that up to 50 percent of patients with Hashimoto's have an impaired tolerance to carbohydrates. This means that after consuming carbohydrate-rich foods, their blood sugar goes up too high, too quickly. This leads to a rapid, sometimes excessive release of insulin. These insulin surges can cause low blood sugar, which can cause unpleasant symptoms such as nervousness, lightheadedness, anxiety, and fatigue. Beyond unpleasantness, this reaction is a huge stressor for the adrenals.

Before I balanced my blood sugar, I would get "hangry" (hungry + angry) multiple times per day as the high-carbohydrate foods I was eating were making me have huge blood sugar swings. What I didn't know is that these swings were also weakening my adrenals and causing a spike in my thyroid antibodies.

I wasn't aware that I had blood sugar issues when I was first diagnosed (despite being a self-admitted sugar addict). I was thin, so I

The Carbohydrate and Fat Myth

During pharmacy school we learned about nutrient requirements in our first-year biochemistry course. I was shocked to learn that carbohydrates were not a required nutrient, while fat was required for normal cell function. Based on my previous nutrition "knowledge" gathered from store displays, the USDA Food Guide Pyramid, and Subway commercials, I was led to believe that carbohydrates were essential and fats were unhealthy.

I am sure I was not the only person misled by the "low fat" labeling of foods and the prominent placement of carbohydrates as the base of the Food Guide Pyramid. Fortunately, the new USDA MyPlate no longer encourages people to eat the equivalent of one loaf of bread on a daily basis. However, people with Hashimoto's need to refine their diet even further. While different diets may have benefits for people with various conditions, in the case of Hashimoto's, a diet lower in carbohydrates seems to work best.

A 2016 study published in the journal *Drug Design, Development and Therapy* found a reduction in weight and thyroid antibodies in thyroid patients over the course of just three weeks of implementing a low-carbohydrate diet. While the standard American diet consists of 50 percent carbohydrates, 15 percent protein, and 35 percent fat, the proportions in the study included 12 to 15 percent carbohydrates, 50 to 60 percent protein, and 25 to 30 percent fat. I have seen some clients benefit from a similar ratio as in the study, as well as a ratio of higher fat and lower protein in others. Regardless of the optimal protein vs. fat ratio for you, I do recommend lowering carbohydrate intake.

thought that it meant that I was healthy. I recently had this conversation with a client who thought he was in the clear to eat sugar because he did not have diabetes. But you see, diabetes takes many years to develop and is an advanced form of physiologic maladaptation. Subtle signs like impaired carbohydrate tolerance, insulin resistance, blood sugar swings, and hypoglycemia may be seen for many years before one develops diabetes, but these signs and symptoms are usually not picked up by conventional tests.

Chronic Inflammation

Chronic inflammation is associated with most autoimmune conditions, especially Hashimoto's thyroiditis, which is essentially inflammation of the thyroid gland. Inflammation can trigger adrenal fatigue as well as an autoimmune cascade.

Inflammation signals the release of cortisol in the body and can result in hypersecretion or depletion of cortisol, which are two ways that the adrenals can dysfunction. Reducing inflammation in the body will help to improve outcomes in most cases of Hashimoto's. Chronic inflammation can be caused by diet, emotions, injuries, gut flora, and low-grade infections. Diet-wise, chronic inflammation occurs when people eat pro-inflammatory foods like conventionally raised meats, processed foods, and foods they are sensitive to.

The Four-Week Adrenal Recovery Protocol

Recovering from adrenal fatigue involves addressing nutrients that may be depleted in long-term adrenal dysfunction, balancing the blood sugar, getting plenty of rest, removing reactive foods and infections, and reducing the stress in our lives! Taking adaptogens and replenishing levels of B vitamins, vitamin C, magnesium, and selenium will also be an important part of the protocol.

All people with adrenal issues will benefit from the Fundamental Adrenal Recovery Protocol. This protocol can be started right after taking the adrenal assessment, without the need for saliva test results.

The five steps of the Adrenal Recovery Protocol will look like this:

1. Rest.
2. De-stress.
3. Reduce inflammation.
4. Balance the blood sugar.
5. Replenish nutrients and add adaptogens.

As you get ready to begin this recovery plan, I think it's important to also consider some insight from some of my Root Cause Rebels who've been where you are today. When I surveyed over two thousand of them about what made them feel better and what made them feel worse, here's what they had to say:

MAKES ME FEEL BETTER

Sleeping 74%
Spending time with loved ones 73%
Being in nature 71%
Walking 66%
Massage 62%
Reading 61%
Sitting on a beach 60%
Being warm 60%
Hugging 49%
Yoga 39%

MAKES ME FEEL WORSE

Lack of sleep 95%
Being stressed out 93%
Being around negative people 76%
Fighting with loved ones 73%
Lack of sunshine 66%

Cold weather 53%

Being in traffic 41%

Winter 38%

Intense exercise 37%

Drinking alcohol 35%

Root Cause Reflection: What Makes You Feel Better?

1. Write out a list of what makes you feel better and what makes you feel worse.
2. Make a plan for doing more of what makes you better, and less of what makes you worse. Write it down.

Looking over these lists, I can tell you that the feel-better list is full of adrenal boosters, while the feel-worse column is filled with adrenal busters. Alcohol, much like sugar, can make someone feel temporarily better but is an overall adrenal buster. I encourage you to keep these lists in mind as you work through the Adrenal Recovery Protocol and to try to focus on doing more things that make you feel better, and fewer things that make you feel worse.

Step 1: Rest

First and foremost, the most fundamental recommendation of all for adrenal health is sleep! If you are serious about overcoming adrenal fatigue, I suggest to committing to a solid ten to twelve hours of sleep each night for at least fourteen days. Let go of any guilt, and quiet the voice inside your head that's trying to convince you that you're being lazy and self-indulgent. If you have Hashimoto's and adrenal fatigue, you are in need of care, and you need and deserve the rest. Taking this time for yourself will help you create long-term, even permanent, recovery. Of course, this amount of extra sleep may not be possible for a number of reasons. I urge you to try your best to prioritize sleep regardless of the situation. If you can't get to ten hours, get as close as you can to that amount. Here are some insights that will improve the quality of your sleep.

I recommend getting blackout curtains, and if possible, going to bed between 9:00 and 10:00 P.M. and staying in bed until 9:00 A.M. Thyroid and adrenal expert Dr. Alan Christianson reports that we get our most quality sleep before midnight, and Dr. James L. Wilson, another adrenal expert, has noted that the hours between 7:00 and 9:00 A.M. seem to be the most regenerative for most with adrenal fatigue. In tracking my sleep and the sleep of my clients (I like the ŌURA ring for sleep tracking) with adrenal dysfunction, I've found my data seems to echo these hours—deep sleep has been shown to take place early in the night, between the hours of 10:00 P.M. and 2:00 A.M., while REM sleep seems to peak between 5:00 A.M. and 9:00 A.M.

According to Dr. Michael Breus, aka "The Sleep Doctor":

Stages 3 and 4 sleep (known collectively as deep sleep) are the most physically restorative sleep. This is where the bulk of growth hormone is produced, and that helps repair and rebuild muscles as well as tell the brain where to distribute fat and glucose. REM sleep is the mentally restorative sleep. Here is where your brain moves information from your short-term memory to your long-term memory. Your brain is taking all the information you collected during the day, filtering out the unnecessary stuff, and then organizing the pertinent information for retrieval later.

Kick the Caffeine

If you haven't already cut caffeine in the Liver Support Protocol, this is a reminder that in order to heal, you will need to kick your caffeine habit. You may think that caffeine is helping you stay awake and productive, but it is likely sabotaging your health. Drinking even small amounts of caffeine in the form of black tea can be problematic for compromised adrenals and can prevent you from getting the restorative and healing sleep you need. Please refer to chapter 4 for strategies to break your caffeine habit.

Step 2: De-Stress

One of the most common daily challenges for my clients is stress—too much of it, to be exact. It's important to reduce your commitments as much as possible over the next two weeks. If you can go on vacation or have a stay-cation from work, that would be ideal. Any days off would be beneficial. Take some time to lounge, eat good food, and relax. And practice other good relaxation habits: get a massage at least once per week, take hot Epsom salt baths every day, listen to relaxing music, and consider meditation or deep breathing. Think of what you would do at a spa and re-create that same environment in your own life.

While it might seem that managing stress is not something we can improve, there are practices that can make you more stress tolerant and strategies that might even help minimize stress. The key is to become consistent with these stress-reducing techniques. Let's take a look at some of the ones that have been most effective for my clients and me.

Exercise

Many well-meaning individuals who want to be sure that they do everything they possibly can to get their condition better ask me if they should exercise during the protocols. It's a smart question considering that when we're working to heal from Hashimoto's and to support our adrenals, the wrong type of exercise can be counterproductive. At this point in the protocols, my advice is to let your adrenals dictate the optimal amount and type of exercise for your body.

You can tell what stage of adrenal dysfunction you might be in by using this scale from Dr. Alan Christianson, author of *The Adrenal Reset Diet*. He describes the three stages of adrenal dysfunction as follows:

- **Stage 1:** Stressed (edgy, difficulty falling asleep, mental function fast and scattered)
- **Stage 2:** Wired (overwhelmed, difficulty staying asleep, erratic mental function)
- **Stage 3:** Crashed (exhausted, unrefreshing sleep, unable to generate ideas)

Someone with healthy adrenals and even stage 1 adrenal dysfunction may thrive on running, biking, and other cardio types of exercise, which should always be balanced with strength training. However, if you determine that you may be in an advanced stage (stage 2 or especially stage 3), strenuous exercise and cardio-based training, even vigorous walking, could make you feel worse. Regardless of which stage you are in, you can benefit from relaxing exercises such as stretching and muscle training.

Muscle-training activities will be important because they can help restore balance between the breaking down (catabolic) and building up (anabolic) processes that occur in the body. In a healthy person, this balance is typically maintained. However, in a person with adrenal dysfunction, a catabolic process can take over, resulting in the breaking down of too much tissue.

To get started, I recommend gentle, muscle-building exercises like yoga, Pilates, or weight training one to three times per week. As you work to incorporate exercise, be sure to get plenty of rest. Here's a little more about the recommended types of exercise:

- **Yoga:** A gentle exercise with a big focus on breathing, mindfulness, and stretching, yoga is an excellent exercise for stress reduction.

- **Pilates:** This exercise works to recondition and realign the body, improving our posture and the way we move our muscles, leading to a gradual strengthening and toning of the body. Some experts believe that bad posture, such as hunching over, may contribute to thyroid issues. In theory, this could be true, as bad posture can put pressure on the thyroid gland. Pilates can help with fixing posture.
- **Weight training:** Lifting weights helps to build up muscle, putting the body into the anabolic buildup mode.

As a general rule, you should only do exercise that makes you feel better. If you feel more tired after exercise, this means that your adrenals are not yet ready for it. I've had clients who've worn themselves down further by overdoing it with exercise in the hopes that it would help with weight loss.

One such client was Lindsay, who was a busy mom and carved out two hours each day to walk outside or on the treadmill. She was dealing with fatigue, brain fog, and irritability, but she was especially frustrated with her weight, and neither her thyroid medications nor dietary changes seemed to be helping.

When I reviewed Lindsey's case, I discovered that she had some dietary adjustments that she needed to make, but I found that her adrenals needed some rest as well—her adrenal saliva test showed that she was in stage 3 fatigue. I recommended that she stop her walking regimen for one month, spend more time resting and practicing self-care, and take adrenal adaptogens to support her adrenal hormones. After sticking to my suggestions for one month, Lindsey reported that she felt happier and healthier, and she had lost seven pounds without feeling hungry or counting calories.

Just like with Lindsey, I recommend that you make sure you're doing only adrenal-appropriate exercises. As you can see in her case, even too much walking was proving problematic. Adrenal-friendly exercises should provide more energy and a sense of accomplishment, and make you feel like you could do the exercise all over again.

Think Positive

Thinking positive thoughts and practicing meditation can shift your body into rest-digest-and-heal mode. In essence, positive thoughts and relaxation send your body messages to promote healing. Even pausing to practice yogic breathing can lead to increased feelings of calm. One of my favorite yogic-breathing techniques is the 4–7–8, where you breathe in for a count of four, hold your breath for a count of seven, and then breathe out for a count of eight.

Émile Coué was a French pharmacist and psychologist who found that positive thoughts could improve healing. Positive thoughts can come in the form of affirmations, which you can repeat throughout the day. Émile Coué's original mantra is "Every day in every way I am getting better and better."

Here are some additional affirmations I've found helpful:

"I love myself."
"I am powerful."
"I am healing."
"I am loved."
"The world is a safe and beautiful place."
"I am beautiful."

I also recommend practicing mindfulness as a way of diminishing stress. This means pausing and truly being present in the moment—taking time to notice all of the beauty, kindness, and good things that are present in the world. And if at first you don't see it, try looking a bit harder—you might just be surprised as you suddenly become aware of the beauty in the trees or the kindness of strangers, even the flowers on the side of the road that you've driven so many times before.

Other Ways to Reduce Stress

Additional strategies for de-stressing that you may find helpful include reading self-help books, practicing gratitude, listening to spa music, meditating, organizing, decluttering, laughing, getting a pet, walking, knitting, and journaling.

If you are someone who always feels like you are running behind, forgetting things, and generally failing at life, taking a day to "plan" your life can be very liberating and uplifting. Look for redundancies in your schedule, opportunities to let go of responsibilities and delegate, and ways to systematize or automate tasks when possible. Perhaps you can do all of your week's shopping on Mondays, batch cook on Tuesdays, and pay your recurring bills with automatic payments. It may help to plan downtime as well, to give yourself healthy boundaries of how many responsibilities you can take on.

I've also found scheduling "personal management time" on a weekly basis to be crucial. Whether it's one weeknight after work or during the weekend, take four hours for yourself without any responsibilities—do what you want to do, not what you should do. Take that time to do whatever your heart desires, whether it's catching a movie by yourself, meeting a friend for lunch, shopping, or going to a day spa.

Use these ideas as a starting point, and take some time to identify strategies to shift your body into a state of relaxing, digesting, and healing.

Step 3: Reduce Inflammation

I wish I could give you a magic pill to eliminate the inflammation in your body, but as you may have guessed, reducing inflammation is not an immediate process. Instead, it happens in a gradual process, but we can take steps to encourage it.

We already began some work on inflammation in the Fundamental Liver Support Protocol, where we took away the three most inflammatory foods and added supplements that reduce inflammation. During the Fundamental Adrenal Recovery Protocol, we will further refine our foods by following the Root Cause Paleo Diet and work on reducing inflammatory thoughts. We will also continue working on inflammation throughout the Fundamental Gut Balance Protocol, where we will tackle additional triggers and add targeted anti-inflammatory supplements. For some people, these strategies will be enough to reduce inflammation. For others, one or more of the Advanced Protocols will be needed.

Root Cause Paleo Diet

The Root Cause Paleo Diet includes nuts, seeds, meats, eggs, vegetables, and fruit, and it excludes all processed foods as well as grains. This diet is designed to lower your intake of inflammatory foods and increase your intake of anti-inflammatory foods, including high-quality animal-based proteins, which will help your body repair itself. While the Root Cause Paleo Diet has origins in the traditional Paleo diet, a diet designed to reflect what our ancestors ate, I've made strategic modifications to ensure that it specifically benefits people with Hashimoto's. For example, pea protein is controversial in the traditional Paleo diet, but it will be included here because it's a hypoallergenic protein for people with Hashimoto's and is well tolerated by most.

THE ROOT CAUSE PALEO DIET EXCLUDES:

Caffeine

Dairy

Grains

Hot peppers

Legumes (except green beans and pea protein)

Seaweed

Sugar

THE ROOT CAUSE PALEO DIET INCLUDES:

All fruits

All meats

All vegetables (except cayenne peppers)

Eggs

Nuts

Pea protein (try the Root Cause Green Smoothie, recipe on page 119)

Hydrolyzed beef protein (try the Root Cause Build Smoothie, recipe on page 178)

Seeds

Additional Guidelines

. You may be surprised that I am recommending a diet that contains meat, as you may have heard that eating meat is inflammatory. This is true for conventionally raised animals, which have high levels of pro-inflammatory omega-6 fatty acids, but meat plays an important repair role in the body, and naturally raised animals have the optimal ratio of anti-inflammatory omega-3 fatty acids for human consumption. Look for grass-fed, pasture-raised, wild-caught, and free-range options.

In addition to the standard Paleo diet guideline, I've found that avoiding hot peppers (they lead to leaky gut), all dairy (even butter and ghee), and seaweeds (due to iodine content and immune-modulating potential) and eating more vegetables than on the traditional Paleo diet lead to improved outcomes for most people.

The inclusion of hydrolyzed beef protein for smoothies (see page 178 for recipe) provides a nutrient-dense snack or breakfast and alleviates fatigue due to helping with digestion and nutrition absorption.

I'd love to share some printable meal plans, recipes, and shopping lists with you so you can get started. Please go to www.thyroidpharmacist.com/action to get access!

Step 4: Balance the Blood Sugar

Food deprivation and blood sugar imbalances place unnecessary stress on the body. If you have impaired glucose tolerance, hypoglycemia, and the early start of insulin resistance, as most people with

My Adrenal Balancing Act

As someone who has gone from being a public health pharmacist with health struggles to a health activist, author, and entrepreneur, my workload has greatly increased. Not to mention my capacity to do more. When I was sick, I was too tired to follow any of my dreams. Once I got my energy back, I began to make up for lost time … and ended up burning the candle at both ends. I wrote and published a book and started a blog and a Facebook page. I then found that I was spending all of my free time writing for my blog, interacting with people on Facebook, working with people with Hashimoto's, and speaking on radio shows and online summits as an expert on reversing Hashimoto's.

I also began to travel a lot more. My husband and I decided to live in Europe for a year, and I left my job as a clinical pharmacist. I was excited to live in Europe and loved traveling to different countries every few weeks. I got a chance to visit Spain, Poland, Greece, Germany, and many other countries while living abroad. The downside was that I was constantly jet-lagged, fell out of my routine, and stopped going to yoga. I began to become dependent on caffeine and often stayed up late working on projects. I always thought, *It's for a good cause—I'm helping people with Hashimoto's!*

But I forgot that even though I may have felt better, that didn't make me superhuman. And despite the fact that I was eating an excellent diet, I eventually slipped back into adrenal fatigue and had to restart adrenal supplements and work my way back to health … again.

Now, to maintain my adrenal health, I have realized that I need the following in my life:

- **Healthy boundaries:** Making self-care a priority, setting limits for myself, and learning to say no help me stay centered amid numerous opportunities and requests.
- **Social interaction:** As a natural extrovert, I strive for connecting with people and get energy from spending time with others. Working in solitude on mundane tasks day in and day out is my personal definition of hell and puts unneeded stress on my well-being.
- **Yoga or Pilates practice:** Going to yoga or Pilates one to three times per week helps me to balance out my mind and body.
- **Mindfulness practice:** This makes me feel relaxed and peaceful.
- **Regular bedtime:** Going to sleep at a decent hour helps me to be rested.
- **Caffeine avoidance:** Caffeine makes me think I have superpowers and causes me to stay up even when I'm tired and should be resting.
- **Daily Epsom salt baths:** These play a big part in helping me de-stress.
- **Weekly Izabella management sessions:** I spend at least four hours each week where I ignore every responsibility I have and just do something I feel like doing. For me, it's usually something like getting a massage, browsing at clothing stores, or doing something girly.
- **Vacations:** A vacation is always helpful if you want to unwind (I think you'd agree that none of us take these as often as we would like!).
- **Supplements:** If I am particularly stressed or working under a deadline, I will take extra adrenal support supplements.

Hashimoto's do, you can make a big difference in your symptoms as well as slow or halt your progression toward diabetes and Hashimoto's by adjusting your nutrition. Balancing my blood sugar made a big difference for me, helping with my anxiety levels and reducing my thyroid antibodies.

To help balance your blood sugar over the next two weeks, I want you to focus on eating fats and proteins, especially for your morning meal, and when you are hungry, focus on making sure you eat and that you eat until you are full. This will reset your body's thinking that food is scarce and will reduce the stress you have put on your body.

Before you start the Adrenal Recovery Protocol, I recommend taking some time to plan out two weeks' worth of meals and batch cook as many as you can. Once you start following the dietary recommendations outlined here, you should notice that you will feel calmer and better within a week or so. To help keep track of how you're feeling, start journaling your symptoms and how they change as you modify your diet.

How Food Impacts Your Blood Sugar

The best measure for gauging how food impacts your blood sugar is to consider the glycemic index. The glycemic index is a measure of how quickly food is converted into glucose (blood sugar) and then becomes assimilated into our bodies. You can also think of it as the burn rate of food because it essentially represents how quickly we burn the fuel we receive from these foods. Rather than trying to learn every food's individual glycemic index, it's simpler to think of it in terms of categories:

- **Carbohydrates:** Sugars and starches have a very quick burn rate. The carbohydrates become assimilated very quickly into our bodies, which causes a rapid and high spike in blood sugar. After eating carbohydrates, we become hungry again after less than an hour.

- **Fats and proteins:** These have a slower burn rate. They become assimilated into our bodies more slowly and gradually, and they don't raise blood sugar levels as quickly. They also keep us full longer. Assuming we've eaten enough calories to feel full, we will be hungry again two to three hours after eating protein, four hours after eating fat.

The following quick reference chart can make balancing your blood sugar much easier. Remember, the foods that keep you fuller longer are better for your blood sugar:

FOOD AND HUNGER GUIDE

Type of Food	Time Until You Are Hungry Again
Carbohydrate	45 minutes–1 hour
Protein	2–3 hours
Fat	4 hours

In general, I recommend limiting carbohydrates in preference of eating fats, proteins, and veggies. When you do eat carbohydrates, such as sweet potatoes, fruits, and the occasional gluten-free grain, always combine them with fat or protein. Never exceed a 2:1 carb-to-protein ratio. This will ensure the overall glycemic load of your meal stays low.

Eating a low glycemic index diet helps with feeling fuller longer and improves cholesterol levels, blood sugar levels, cognitive performance, energy, and complexion. It also reduces your risk of developing diabetes, heart disease, and some cancers and promotes weight loss for those who are overweight. Many people have also found their moods improve after balancing their blood sugar.

My favorite sources of protein and fat that stabilize blood sugar include the following foods:

- Avocados
- Chia seeds
- Chicken
- Coconut, avocado, or olive oil
- Coconut milk
- Duck fat
- Eggs (if not sensitive)
- Egg white protein (if not sensitive)
- Grass-fed beef
- Hydrolyzed beef protein
- Lamb
- Nuts (except peanuts)
- Olives
- Pea protein
- Pork
- Salmon
- Sardines
- Seeds like pumpkin
- Tallow
- Turkey
- White fish

I recommend that you have generous amounts of proteins and fats with each meal. Adding in fiber may be an additional strategy to keep your blood sugar stable.

If you are not sensitive to any of the ingredients listed, starting your day with the Root Cause Smoothie (see page 127) will help you keep blood sugar stable throughout the day.

Habits to Stabilize Your Blood Sugar

There are other dietary strategies you can adopt to help keep your blood sugar balanced. Eating snacks often, especially in the early stages of your blood-sugar-balancing journey, is important, and being sure to eat breakfast within one hour of waking will also help you start the day off on the right foot.

Some good snacks to consider may include nuts, seeds, hard-boiled eggs, Epic bars, homemade beef jerky, sardines, and protein shakes. It's important to note that you may find that you are intolerant to some of these when you do the elimination diet in the Fundamental Gut Balance Protocol, so do not invest in Costco-size jugs just yet.

So what do you eat for your breakfast that you're going to eat within one hour of waking? I recommend that you start the day off with a blood-sugar-balancing smoothie that has a mix of good fat (avocado, chia, egg yolks, coconut oil), protein (egg yolks, hydrolyzed beef protein), and fiber (lettuces, vegetables). The Root Cause Build Smoothie and the Root Cause Green Smoothie (see page 119) are both excellent options for breakfast (and snacks too!). Another good option, which I like to refer to as my Happy Hormones Breakfast, is eggs and bacon + herbal tea with stevia + avocado. This is a perfect alternative to the typical standard American diet breakfast of bagel with cream cheese + orange juice + coffee with sugar.

Root Cause Build Smoothie

½ cup baby carrots

1 avocado

1 cup coconut milk

1 cup greens

2 egg yolks (if tolerated)

1 scoop hydrolyzed beef protein

Add ingredients to a blender and blend thoroughly. You can add water to thin out the consistency, which will make it easier to eat and feel less filling.

How Much Protein Should You Get per Day?

- **Low activity:** Most people with low to moderate amounts of activity should aim for 1.2 g of protein per kilogram of body weight per day.
- **High activity:** Those who are exercising and otherwise active should eat at least 1.2 g per kilogram of body weight per day (that's about 0.5 g per pound).
- **Illness:** Most older adults who have acute or chronic diseases can eat 1.2 to 1.5 g per kilogram of body weight per day. Older people with severe kidney disease (estimated GFR <30 mL/min/1.73 m²), but who are not on dialysis, are an exception to this rule; these individuals may need to limit protein intake.
- **Bodybuilding:** Those lifting heavy weights can eat up to 2 g per kilogram of body weight per day.

As much as there are foods you should eat more of, there are of course items and practices that you should avoid, as these can create unstable blood sugar levels. These are some of the worst blood sugar stressors:

- **Sugar, sweets, and grains:** You likely realize that sweets and sodas are not an ideal food for blood sugar balance. However, if you're anything like me, you may be eating much more sugar than you thought. Wheat and even gluten-free products made with grains like rice, corn, and potatoes can wreak havoc on our blood sugar. This is one of the reasons I advocate a gluten-free and grain-free diet as a starting point for people with Hashimoto's.
- **Fruit and fruit juices:** You may have thought that fruit and fruit juices were healthy snacks—and they are in moderation for the

Root Cause Research Corner: Is Stevia Good or Bad?

Lots of people ask me if stevia is good or bad. Well, it depends! If you are someone who has diabetes, stevia may be helpful, as it has been found to reduce the rise of glucose during glucose tolerance testing and to enhance insulin secretion and insulin utilization.

The medical effects reported with stevia are decreased blood pressure, weight loss, and reduced blood sugar. These are all things that are helpful for people who have high blood sugar, high blood pressure, and are overweight.

But if you are someone in an advanced stage of adrenal fatigue with low blood pressure and hypoglycemia (or are underweight), stevia may worsen your symptoms.

While no studies have been done with stevia on people with hypoglycemia, low blood pressure, or Addison's disease, anecdotally, some individuals have reported that stevia can make their blood sugar drop more, weakening the adrenals.

average healthy person. But for those with stressed adrenals, even the sugar in fruit (and especially in fruit juices) can be too much! Fruit should be limited to one to two servings per day, and fruit juices to a half serving for one month. Once your adrenals have been rebalanced, you will be able to tolerate more fruit.

- **Fasting:** Fasting and the latest intermittent fasting trend are alternative health approaches that have cleansing and healing properties. Unfortunately, they are super stressful on the adrenals. So while some people may benefit from fasting, I've seen that Hashimoto's patients, due to rampant adrenal issues, often feel worse on a fast in the initial stages of healing. This is why I recommend abstaining from fasting during the fundamental healing period.

Step 5: Replenish Nutrients and Add Adaptogens

My supplement protocol for balancing adrenals includes adding adaptogenic herbs, B complex vitamins, and vitamin C as well as selenium and magnesium. These supplements have been found to be safe and effective for most people with Hashimoto's, which is why I do not routinely recommend testing for deficiency before supplementing.

Vitamin C and B vitamins become depleted during high cortisol production and turnover. Deficiencies in pantothenic acid and biotin found in B vitamins in particular have been linked to decreased adrenal function in animals and humans. Potassium, zinc, iron, and magnesium also become depleted with excessive cortisol production and may lead to adrenal fatigue. Replenishing these nutrients helps reverse this course.

Adaptogenic Herbs

Adaptogenic herbs comprise many natural herb products that supplement the body's ability to deal with stressors. In the 1940s pharmacologist Nikolai Lazarev first defined the concept of adaptogens. An adaptogen is a substance that can raise the body's resilience to various types of stress, including physical and emotional stress.

To be considered an adaptogen, an herb must possess several qualities. First, it must be nontoxic to the patient at normal doses. Second, the herb should help the entire body cope with stress. Third, it should help the body to return to normal regardless of how stress is currently affecting the person's functioning. In other words, an adaptogenic herb needs to be able to both tone down overactive systems *and* boost underactive systems in the body. Adaptogens are thought to normalize the hypothalamic-pituitary-adrenal (HPA) axis.

Adaptogenic herbs include ashwagandha, astragalus, reishi mushroom, dang shen, eleuthero, ginseng, jiaogulan, licorice, maca, schisandra, spikenard, and suma. These are examples of herbs that may increase the body's ability to resist stress, and they have been

Switch Up Your Salt!

People with adrenal issues often have salt cravings because of the subclinical electrolyte imbalances caused by adrenal dysfunction (aka the "I just ate a whole bag of chips" syndrome). However, processed salt has been tied to autoimmune disease, and the fortification of salt with iodine is partially responsible for the Hashimoto's epidemic (please refer to my first book, *Hashimoto's Thyroiditis,* for a whole chapter dedicated to this phenomenon). This does not mean that you need to avoid salt. Quite the contrary; I encourage you to consume more salt. But the right kind of salt. Throw away your processed iodized salt and switch it for non-iodized sea salt (gray or pink is best), which is filled with nutrients and the yummy salt our body craves!

Add ample salt to your satisfaction to your foods, and add a teaspoon of sea salt into a glass of warm water to drink throughout the day for fluid balance support.

helpful in relieving adrenal dysfunction when used in combination with vitamins and minerals.

I've also found Yogi licorice tea to be a gentle adrenal tonic (avoid if you have high blood pressure). Adding some maca root to your smoothies may also be helpful. I formulated Rootcology Adrenal Support, and another high-quality option is the Daily Stress Formula by Pure Encapsulations.

B Vitamins

B vitamins play an important role in cell metabolism, thyroid function, and adrenal function. They become depleted in stressful situations that often precede the development of autoimmunity.

Four especially important B vitamins are pantothenic acid (B_5), thiamine or benfotiamine (B_1), biotin (B_7), and cobalamin (B_{12}).

A vitamin B complex supplement should be a great start and will be helpful for most people with low energy levels. B vitamins are water-soluble vitamins and do not build up in the body, so the risk for toxicity is almost nonexistent.

In people with severe deficiencies, additional doses of B vitamins may be needed, such as a standalone B_{12} supplement, a biotin supplement, a thiamine supplement, or a methylfolate-containing supplement. I've covered most of these vitamins in greater detail in my first book, *Hashimoto's Thyroiditis*. I'd love to share the "Depletions and Digestion" chapter with you on www.thyroidpharmacist.com/gift.

B_1 (Thiamine)

Thiamine is one of the B vitamins, known as B_1. It has the important roles of converting carbohydrates into energy and aiding with the digestion of proteins and fats. Thiamine is required for proper release of hydrochloric acid in our stomachs, which is needed for proper protein digestion. Most people with Hashimoto's have low stomach acid or do not release any stomach acid. Thiamine supports blood sugar function, adrenals, and can boost our energy levels.

Overt thiamine deficiency is primarily thought to affect alcoholics. However the latest research is suggesting that mild deficiency may exist in people with autoimmune disease and related malabsorption. Thiamine is an important nutrient and is added to fortified processed foods including cereals and breads. As you'll be avoiding processed foods, I recommend supplementing with thiamine. Symptoms of milder forms of thiamine deficiency include fatigue, irritability, depression, brain fog, abdominal discomfort, low blood pressure, low stomach acid, and trouble digesting carbohydrates.

Long-term thiamine deficiency in those who consume any carbohydrates (even fruit) can lead to a buildup of pyruvic acid, which is a by-product of glucose metabolism, and can lead to mental fog,

Choosing the Most Optimal Form of B Vitamin

B Vitamin Number	Name	Optimal Form
B_1	Thiamine	Thiamine HCl or benfotiamine
B_2	Riboflavin	Riboflavin-5'-phosphate
B_3	Niacin	Niacinamide
B_5	Pantothenic acid	D-calcium pantothenate
B_6	Pyridoxine	Pyridoxal-5-phosphate
B_7	Biotin	D-biotin
B_8	Inositol	Myo-inositol
B_9	Folate	Methylfolate, Metafolin, or NatureFolate
B_{12}	Cobalamin	Methylcobalamin

difficulty breathing, and heart damage. Those on low-carbohydrate diets are at a smaller risk of the buildup of pyruvic acid and may not have any symptoms except for fatigue.

The recommended daily allowance for thiamine is only 1.1 mg for women over nineteen years of age and may not meet the needs of those who are on a grain-free diet and have malabsorption issues (very common with autoimmune disease). Researchers in Italy found that taking a 600 mg dose of thiamine relieved fatigue in women with Hashimoto's who were already taking thyroid medication. I have seen excellent results with thiamine as well as benfotiamine, a thiamine derivative.

I can't tell you how many readers have run up to me at conferences to give me a hug or thank me for my blog post on thiamine, which helped turn their fatigue around.

Remember, 600 mg is a megadose of thiamine, so you will likely have to take multiple tablets or capsules to get to that target (you won't find a sufficient dose of thiamine in most B complex formulas).

Root Cause Research Corner: A Caution for Cancer Patients—Thiamine Might Not Be for You

While thiamine in the recommended doses is extremely safe for most people, it should not be taken by people with advanced cancers. This is because thiamine is necessary for cell replication, and it's possible that cancer cells will steal the body's reserves of thiamine and use it to proliferate themselves. Providing just enough thiamine to correct the thiamine deficiency can help the tumor grow (the thiamine goes to the tumor instead of us), while megadoses of thiamine actually inhibit tumor growth. If you have a thiamine deficiency and cancer, I would advise you to work with a cancer specialist.

Unfortunately, standard lab tests for thiamine deficiency will not show if someone is mildly deficient—they will only show a severe deficiency of thiamine. If you've been struggling with fatigue, low stomach acid, carbohydrate intolerance, low blood pressure, and your adrenals, you may benefit from a trial of thiamine.

Vitamin C

Vitamin C is an essential vitamin for supporting adrenal function. I recommend doses of 500 mg to 3,000 mg per day, as tolerated.

Selenium

Selenium deficiency has widely been recognized as an environmental trigger for Hashimoto's. Selenium plays a very important role in thyroid function, acting as catalyst to convert the inactive T4 to the biologically active T3, and protecting thyroid cells from oxidative damage that occurs during the production of thyroid hormones.

Root Cause Reflection: Hashimoto's Anxiety

We know that stress, anxiety, and being high-strung can contribute to adrenal issues, but it's a two-way street. Many of my readers and clients report that the onset of Hashimoto's changed their previously calm and laid-back demeanor. One reader wrote: "After my Hashimoto's diagnosis, all of a sudden I found myself with panic attacks and anxiety. This was not me. I went from a comfortable social butterfly to a constantly anxious person who could barely speak up in work meetings. It's like all of a sudden I couldn't cope with anything!"

In stage 2 and beyond in Hashimoto's, the thyroid is under attack by the immune system. As thyroid cells are broken down, they release thyroid hormones into the bloodstream. This causes thyroid hormone surges, or a transient hyperthyroidism. This excess amount of thyroid hormone can make us extremely anxious, irritable, and on edge. This is one symptom that is commonly attributed to Graves' disease but can also happen in Hashimoto's.

I know how awful anxiety can feel, and so I'm really excited to share that there is a way out. You don't have to feel this way forever. Everyone is different, but two of the things that have worked wonders for my clients and me are the following: supplementing with selenium in the morning and magnesium citrate at bedtime, and balancing the blood sugar with nutrition.

Do you struggle with anxiety?

Did you realize this symptom could be due to Hashimoto's?

If you were less anxious, how would that improve your life?

Selenium deficiency can occur when we have gut issues because of malabsorption from damage to the small intestine.

Supplemental selenium has been found to reduce Hashimoto's antibodies and symptoms, improve Graves' disease health outcomes, and reduce the incidence of postpartum thyroiditis when taken during pregnancy.

Selenium has a narrow therapeutic index, and doses of under 100 mcg may not be sufficient for improving Hashimoto's symptoms and markers, while doses in excess of 800 mcg per day can be toxic. Numerous studies have shown that a dosage of 200 mcg of selenium methionine per day has been found to reduce thyroid antibodies in clinical trials—in some studies selenium cut thyroid antibodies in half within three months. This is why I always recommend taking a selenium supplement in lieu of getting selenium from Brazil nuts. While it's true that Brazil nuts are a rich source of selenium, the selenium content varies in the nuts based on where the nuts were grown, thus a person may inadvertently consume insufficient or toxic amounts of selenium.

In my experience, a dose of 200 to 400 mcg per day of selenium methionine can help people with Hashimoto's reduce thyroid antibodies and feel more calm, and can also improve energy levels and hair regrowth.

I don't routinely recommend testing for selenium levels; rather, I've found that selenium supplementation in the range of 200 to 400 mcg per day is generally safe and effective for most people with Hashimoto's.

Magnesium

I already discussed the use of magnesium in the Liver Support Protocol, and I recommend continuing this important supplement throughout the Adrenal Recovery and Gut Balance Protocols. As this nutrient is depleted by stress and is often difficult to obtain from foods, most people will benefit from long-term supplementation.

Next Steps and Roadblocks

Inadequate rest, emotional stress, blood sugar imbalances, and inflammation are the primary drivers of adrenal dysfunction. In this chapter, I've outlined a protocol that addresses those triggers and that most people with Hashimoto's and adrenal issues will be able to follow and benefit from. Further adrenal boosting interventions will be introduced in the final Fundamental Protocol, the Gut Balance Protocol, where we will add inflammation-reducing supplements, further optimize nutrition, and address dysbiosis and impaired digestion (which also contribute to inflammation).

Following the Adrenal Recovery Protocol for four weeks will help most people with adrenal dysfunction feel significantly better, and you will see further improvement in your overall and adrenal symptoms as you complete the Gut Balance Protocol. If you continue to have symptoms after completing all the Fundamental Protocols, please refer to chapter 7 to determine additional triggers. You may benefit from further interventions for balancing the stress response, such as adrenal saliva testing, taking adrenal hormones or glandulars, or addressing traumatic stress with targeted therapies. Don't worry, everything done during the Fundamental Protocols will help you feel better and will build the foundation for further healing. Let's move on to addressing your gut health next!

ADRENAL SUPPLEMENT OVERVIEW

Preferred Products	Description
Adrenal Support by Rootcology, Daily Stress Formula by Pure Encapsulations, or Adrenotone by Designs for Health	A mixture of adaptogenic herbs, vitamins, minerals, and amino acids to support the adrenals.
	Blends containing ashwagandha should be avoided in people with nightshade reactions.*

Preferred Products	Description
B-Complex Plus by Pure Encapsulations	B vitamins, especially pantothenic acid (B_5) and thiamine (B_1), support proper adrenal function, and methylcobalamin (B_{12}) supports energy function. Some individuals may also benefit from sublingual B_{12} formulations.
BenfoMax 600 mg by Pure Encapsulations	Thiamine and benfotiamine support energy levels in people with Hashimoto's. Doses of 600 mg per day are recommended.
Vitamin C by NOW Foods	Vitamin C is an essential vitamin for proper adrenal function. Doses of 500–3,000 mg per day are helpful for adrenal function. Reduce dose if diarrhea occurs.
Selenium by Pure Encapsulations	Selenium is a nutrient that has been found to reduce thyroid antibodies and anxiety. Doses of 200–400 mcg of selenium methionine are recommended.
Magnesium (citrate) by Pure Encapsulations	Magnesium supports healthy DHEA levels and promotes a restful sleep. The citrate salt helps promote bowel movements. Reduce dose or switch to magnesium glycinate if diarrhea occurs.

*See more information on nightshade sensitivity on page 105.

6

Gut Balance Protocol

Welcome to the third and final Fundamental Protocol, which is designed to restore balance to your gut. The first two protocols have likely helped you stabilize hormones, address chemical sensitivities, and minimize—even get rid of—joint pains, rashes, brain fog, mood swings, and fatigue. In other words, hopefully you are already feeling significantly better! Now as we get to the gut, we will work to repair your damaged intestinal lining and imbalanced gut flora, which can be the source of symptoms such as acid reflux, bloating, irritable bowel syndrome (IBS), anxiety, and more. Get ready for some targeted gut love (yes, your gut needs love too) and, better yet, for the improvements you'll experience on the other side of this protocol.

Understanding Leaky Gut

We've discussed that intestinal permeability is a factor in every case of autoimmune disease, with Hashimoto's of course being no different. Otherwise known as leaky gut, intestinal permeability is defined by gaps in the gut lining that can develop and allow for irritating molecules and substances to escape into the bloodstream. According to research from Dr. Alessio Fasano, every person with an autoimmune disorder has some degree of leaky gut.

While it might sound unpleasant or unsolvable, intestinal permeability actually offers those of us with autoimmunity a great opportunity for healing. We know that autoimmunity needs a combination of the right genes, the right triggers, and intestinal permeability to manifest itself (referred to in the functional medicine world as the three-legged stool of autoimmunity). Of those three factors, our genes represent a relatively fixed factor, and triggers may be tough to identify with certainty, but intestinal permeability ... this is something we can work with! I was so excited when I first learned about leaky gut because it provided me with a clear area of focus.

The discovery that intestinal permeability is a factor in autoimmune thyroid disease represented a major breakthrough in the understanding of the condition. Unfortunately, you're not likely to come across an endocrinologist who will recommend addressing intestinal permeability as part of your treatment. Our current mainstream medical system is very fragmented and treats each organ as though it was living by itself in a vacuum. The connection between gluten and gut infections in Hashimoto's has been published in well-established gastroenterology medical journals, but most endocrinologists simply do not read those journals. They instead depend on endocrinology journals, which focus primarily on improved diagnostic and surgical methods for the thyroid gland.

Thankfully, we have the world of natural and functional medicine to turn to when we're looking for more progressive, open-minded professionals. In these areas of medicine, the concepts that all disease begins in the gut and that leaky gut is a common denominator have been widely accepted, and the protocols focused on healing the gut have produced numerous success stories.

Intestinal permeability made a lot of sense to me because I had many of the symptoms including bloating, stomach pains, IBS, and acid reflux. These same symptoms are commonly experienced by people with Hashimoto's, although not everyone with intestinal permeability or Hashimoto's will have these symptoms. Some may have no apparent gut symptoms at all, but their gut function might need to be addressed nonetheless.

Interestingly, fetal origin of the thyroid gland is the same as the stomach, digestive tract, and tongue—thus we can consider thyroid cells as digestive tract cells. A rare birth defect can even place a fully functioning thyroid gland that makes thyroid hormones at the base of the tongue instead of inside of the neck. The "tongue thyroid" can even develop Hashimoto's and become enlarged. This shared cellular origin may be another reason why improving digestive function often leads to a significant improvement in thyroid symptoms.

The Million-Dollar Question: Why Does the Gut Become Permeable? (And How Do We Heal It?)

The healthy human intestine has the important role of acting as both a barrier and a filter through selectively closing and opening intestinal tight junctions, depending on the need. The healthy intestine allows for nutrients to be absorbed, and blocks the absorption of toxins and pathogens. In the case of autoimmune disease, the gut becomes too permeable, so potentially problematic substances get absorbed. Various factors have the ability to modulate the intestinal tight junctions, and the key to restoring their function is to eliminate these triggers. Here are some of the factors that contribute to increased intestinal permeability:

- Adrenal fatigue
- Alcohol
- Capsaicin (in peppers and paprika)
- Dysbiosis
- Enzyme deficiencies
- Food sensitivities
- Gluten
- Gut infections

- Nonsteroidal anti-inflammatory drugs (NSAIDs)
- Nutrient depletions
- Psychological stress
- Small intestinal bacterial overgrowth (SIBO)
- Sinus infections, mouth infections
- Strenuous exercise
- Stress
- Surgery or trauma
- Toxins

While there are numerous factors that can cause intestinal permeability, the most common ones are stress, food sensitivities, nutrient deficiencies, deficiency in digestive enzymes, an imbalance of gut bacteria, and intestinal infections. We've already addressed a few of these in the first two protocols: you've taken steps to improve your stress response and paid attention to some common food sensitivities and nutrient deficiencies (and you should continue as many of those interventions as you can for three to six months). In this chapter, we will focus on uncovering additional food sensitivities, correcting previously unaddressed nutrient deficiencies, and balancing enzymes and gut bacteria. Intestinal infections, which often require testing and targeted therapies, will be covered in the Advanced Protocols.

By following the interventions in this chapter, you will start seeing a reduction of any residual symptoms you may have (especially gut-related symptoms), and your thyroid antibody levels should also show a decline within six weeks of these interventions. If you don't see an improvement after six weeks and don't see a full resolution of symptoms after completing all the Fundamental Protocols, you likely have additional triggers, such as a gut infection, that will need further investigation and intervention. You will want to continue the protocol as you work to identify additional triggers. Don't despair if you find you're in this latter group—doing the

GUT HEALTH ASSESSMENT
Mark which symptoms apply to you.

☐ I have an autoimmune condition.
☐ I have gas.
☐ I have food sensitivities.
☐ I have irritable bowel syndrome.
☐ I have fewer than one bowel movement per day.
☐ I have hard-to-pass stools.
☐ I have diarrhea.
☐ I have constipation.
☐ I have stomach cramps.
☐ I tend to have undigested food in my stools.
☐ I need to take laxatives to have bowel movements.
☐ I have taken antacids (Pepto-Bismol, Maalox, Tums, and so on) more than once in the past year.
☐ I have taken acid-blocking medications like Pepcid, famotidine, Prevacid, omeprazole, Zantac, Nexium, or Prilosec in the last five years.
☐ I have taken antibiotics for more than two weeks.
☐ I have taken more than three courses of antibiotics in the last ten years before my symptoms started.
☐ I have taken a steroid medication like prednisone for more than two weeks in the last ten years before my symptoms started.
☐ I have taken the birth control pill.
☐ I take over-the-counter pain relievers like ibuprofen, Aleve, Advil, or naproxen on a regular basis.
☐ I have skin rashes, acne, or hives.
☐ I have seasonal or environmental allergies.
☐ I have a swollen, patchy, or coated tongue.
☐ I feel bloated after eating or experience gas or belching.
☐ I have anal itching.
☐ I feel nausea after eating.
☐ I have foul-smelling stools.
☐ I have cravings for sweets, alcohol, or carbs.
☐ I drink coffee or alcohol on a daily basis.
☐ I frequently eat out.
☐ I like to eat sushi and meat that is undercooked.

Total number of symptoms: ___

<2: Low Risk
1–2: Intermediate Risk
>3: High Risk

Source: Adapted from Mark Hyman, *The UltraMind Solution: Fix Your Broken Brain by Healing Your Body First* (New York: Scribner, 2008) and *The UltraMind Solution Companion Guide* (Lenox, MA: UltraWellness, 2009).

---

work to support your body over the next six to twelve weeks will accelerate your ability to get rid of any lingering infections, should you have any.

There are four steps to my gut-healing protocol, which will remove some of the triggers I just listed and also help you build a stronger, more resilient gut. Here are the four steps:

1. Remove reactive foods.
2. Supplement with enzymes.
3. Balance the gut flora.
4. Nourish the gut.

Reactive Foods and Food Sensitivities in Hashimoto's

You already learned about the role of food sensitivities in Hashimoto's during the Liver Support Protocol. The Gut Protocol will further refine your diet by eliminating the remaining common reactive foods in Hashimoto's, allowing your gut to heal.

Enzyme Deficiencies, Poorly Digested Proteins, and "Bad" Bacteria

Studies have found that people with Hashimoto's and hypothyroidism often have a deficiency in the digestive enzyme hydrochloric acid, resulting in low levels of stomach acid (hypochlorhydria) or a complete absence of it (achlorhydria). Low stomach acid can make it more difficult to digest proteins, which in turn can lead to increased tiredness. Digestion is one of the biggest energy-requiring processes of our bodies, so when extra metabolic efforts need to be focused there, it can leave you feeling fatigued.

An initial difficulty with digesting proteins can set off a chain-reaction of greater digestive trouble. That's because your weakened digestion might begin to have problems digesting the more complex protein molecules such as those found in gluten, dairy, and soy. When proteins are poorly digested, we are more likely to become sensitive to them, and thus many people with Hashimoto's will be sensitive to gluten, dairy, and soy, among others. This is partially because these proteins are among the most difficult to digest and partially because they are also the most commonly eaten proteins in the standard Western diet. And eventually, you could develop IgG antibodies to these proteins, which are the very same antibodies that target the thyroid gland in autoimmune disease. When someone continues to eat these proteins, the immune system attack becomes upregulated as the influx of poorly digested proteins triggers the immune system to make more of these types of antibodies.

Making a bad situation worse, reactive proteins can attach to antibodies, creating what's referred to as circulating immune complexes (CICs). Under normal circumstances, the body can break down CICs using self-made proteolytic enzymes, specific protein-eating enzymes released by the stomach and the duodenum part of the small intestine. However, the proteolytic system can become overwhelmed with too many CICs. As these complexes accumulate, they can contribute to liver congestion, autoimmune disease, and many associated symptoms, such as pain, inflammation, and even heart attacks!

While simply eliminating reactive proteins can help a person to feel much better and reduce the autoimmune attack, leaving low stomach acid unaddressed may leave the door open to additional food sensitivities, including to foods such as grains, eggs, nuts, and seeds.

Poorly digested proteins can also become "food" for opportunistic bacteria that live in our gut. The gut is a delicate environment, which functions best when there is a balanced ratio of probiotic (beneficial) and opportunistic (potentially problematic) bacteria. Imbalanced bacterial flora—when there are more opportunistic than probiotic bacteria—is seen as the root cause in many autoimmune conditions, and most people with Hashimoto's have been shown to have imbalanced bacterial flora. This bacterial imbalance is also considered a contributor to intestinal permeability. Over the past few years, I've seen that my very symptomatic clients tend to have patterns of low diversity, low beneficial bacteria, and elevated levels of opportunistic bacteria. In contrast, clients who feel well tend to have a high diversity, high amount of probiotic bacteria, and low opportunistic bacteria on follow-up tests.

Deficiencies in the hydrochloric acid can additionally make us more susceptible to acquiring gut infections such as *Helicobacter pylori* (*H. pylori*), *Yersinia,* and parasites, which can be a potential root cause of autoimmunity.

You can see that a lot of problems can stem from a deficiency in this important digestive enzyme. And you're probably wondering how it develops. Low stomach acid can result from a number of factors, including nutrient deficiencies (such as in thiamine), a vegetarian or vegan diet, adrenal issues that deplete our chloride stores, and infections like *H. pylori* that neutralize stomach acid to aid their survival. Furthermore, a deficiency of stomach acid leads to various types of anemias, including B_{12} and iron-deficiency anemia because we need stomach acid to extract B_{12} and iron from our protein-containing foods. As you can see, this leads to a vicious cycle that results in hair loss, fatigue, food sensitivities, and so on. Many people have been able to improve their levels of ferritin and B_{12} through improving their stomach acid and getting rid of gut infections.

What Is the Best Way to Heal a Leaky Gut?

In order to heal the gut, we need to remove the most common reactive foods for a period of thirty to ninety days and replenish our enzymes to improve digestion and break down CICs. In some cases, enzymes can also help with removing infections by "digesting" the infectious organism or breaking down its protein-containing hiding spot. Simultaneously, we need to supply the body with the nutrients it needs to heal, and we must reestablish balance in our gut flora by encouraging pathogenic bacteria to leave peacefully while replenishing beneficial bacteria.

The Six-Week Gut Balance Protocol

Before you start implementing the steps of this protocol, there are a few prerequisites to gut healing to consider. First, make sure you continue to give yourself the gift of adequate sleep each night, as this will play an important part in healing. Second, you should have also completed the Liver Support and Adrenal Recovery Protocols, which can enhance your results from the Gut Balance Protocol.

The adrenals control the rate at which our gut heals through the cortisol they release, and a deficiency or excess in cortisol can prevent proper gut healing. Inadequate cortisol means we are not controlling inflammation properly, and excess cortisol means we are breaking down the gut barrier for fuel. Supporting the liver first will be important, too, as the multiple immune complexes and impaired gut function often seen in people with autoimmune disease can leave the liver with an excess burden to detoxify.

Lastly, you'll still want to avoid extreme sports and intense physical exertion because this can cause intestinal permeability instead of help correct it—which is one of our primary goals! If you are an extreme athlete, I recommend taking time away from training to fully heal while you are completing these protocols.

The Gut Balance Protocol consists of four steps:

1. Remove reactive foods.
2. Supplement with enzymes.
3. Balance the gut flora.
4. Nourish the gut.

While over the years I've seen many people who have heard about all of the various diets that can be helpful for Hashimoto's, many of them have embarked on these diets without other approaches, and thus the restrictive diets they were eating were only keeping their symptoms at bay temporarily, and many of them hit healing plateaus. After finishing the Gut Balance Protocol, please be sure to look into gut infections and other triggers that may be preventing your proper gut healing.

Step 1: Remove Reactive Foods

At this point, you have excluded the most commonly reactive foods in Hashimoto's, including gluten, dairy, soy, and grains. If you are still having symptoms, especially gut-related symptoms, it's time to step up your diet to the Root Cause Autoimmune Diet, which excludes additional foods that people with Hashimoto's have found reactive, including nuts, nightshades, and eggs.

You're going to follow this diet for six to twelve weeks as you work on healing your gut. You should reevaluate your gut function after six weeks and can start reintroducing foods if all of your gut-related symptoms have resolved. If not, you will need to continue for another six weeks.

The Root Cause Autoimmune Diet

The Root Cause Autoimmune Diet goes a step deeper than the Root Cause Paleo Diet by excluding additional reactive foods.

THE ROOT CAUSE AUTOIMMUNE DIET EXCLUDES:

Caffeine
Dairy

Eggs

Grains

Legumes

Nightshades

Nuts

Seaweed

Seeds

Sugar

THE ROOT CAUSE AUTOIMMUNE DIET INCLUDES:

Fruit, especially coconut

Meat

Olive oil

Shellfish

Vegetables

I know that this may seem like a very short list of foods to enjoy, but I assure you, you will have plenty of delicious choices to eat. Please head over to my website www.thyroidpharmacist.com/action for specially created meal plans, recipes, and shopping lists!

Step 2: Supplement with Enzymes

I recommend two types of enzymes for people with Hashimoto's: digestive enzymes that should be taken with food and proteolytic enzymes that are to be taken on an empty stomach.

Digestive Enzymes

While thiamine can help with increasing stomach acid naturally, betaine with pepsin is another supplement that can be used to raise stomach acid levels. Betaine HCl and pepsin are naturally occurring components of the gastric juices that break down protein bonds in our food to make nutrients and amino acids more bioavailable. They are especially important for proper absorption of protein, calcium, B_{12}, and iron.

Betaine, also known as trimethylglycine, is a naturally occurring amino acid derivative that is isolated from beets, and the acidic HCl version of it promotes stomach acid. Betaine HCl used to be available as an over-the-counter drug, marketed as a stomach acidifier and digestive aid, but it was removed from over-the-counter use in 1993 due to "insufficient evidence of it working" and banished to being a dietary supplement by the FDA (dietary supplement companies cannot make claims of the effectiveness of their products, while drug companies can make specific claims). However, studies done in 2014 did indeed find that betaine HCl can re-acidify gastric pH.

As a side benefit, trimethylglycine can be helpful for breaking down homocysteine, especially in those with the MTHFR gene mutation. Furthermore, it can be a helpful adjunct in depression through increasing endogenous amounts of SAMe, a naturally occurring substance with mood-boosting and pain-relieving properties.

Pepsin is a naturally occurring digestive enzyme (derived from porcine sources in supplements) that breaks proteins into smaller pieces so they can be properly absorbed by the small intestine.

Taking betaine with pepsin while eating protein-containing meals can really support your digestion and boost energy. After beginning to take betaine with pepsin along with my protein-containing meals, the debilitating fatigue I had been dealing with for almost a decade went away practically overnight. I went from sleeping for eleven to twelve hours per night to eight hours simply because I started digesting my food better. In fact, I started writing my first book about overcoming Hashimoto's the morning after I took the right dose of betaine with pepsin—making the connection between my deficiency of stomach acid and Hashimoto's represented that much of an aha moment for me. The restored energy gave me hope that I would be able to devote myself to research and find the root cause of my condition, and that I would be able to share my knowledge to help others.

Unfortunately, low stomach acid may often be misdiagnosed as acid reflux because the symptoms are almost identical. A person diagnosed with acid reflux will typically be placed on acid-blocking medications such as Prilosec, Nexium, or Pepcid, which are known as proton pump inhibitors (PPIs). These medications will do what they're intended to do and suppress stomach acid, which, if you actually have low stomach acid, will only exacerbate nutrient deficiencies and fatigue.

The trick to using betaine with pepsin is figuring out the dose that's right for you, which will take a bit of experimenting.

Start by taking just one capsule (most brands have around 500 mg of betaine and around 20 mg of porcine-derived pepsin per capsule) right after you've eaten a protein-containing meal. Monitor for any reactions, such as a slight burning in your throat. If you do feel a burning in your throat, you do not need the supplement or you did not have enough protein in your meal. Drink a cup of water with a teaspoon of baking soda to relieve any continued burning sensation. If you didn't feel anything, increase your dose to two capsules at the end of your next protein-containing meal.

Then, keep increasing by one capsule until you feel a slight burning or discomfort. Once you've reached this point, you will know that your target dose is one capsule less. For example, if you felt nothing at one capsule, nothing at two capsules, and nothing at three capsules, but a burn at four capsules, your target dose would be three capsules.

This supplement can help fatigue dramatically, and I recommend that you start working on finding your right dose as soon as possible. Hopefully the improvements will be as noticeable for you as they were for me and for many of my clients. Many people with Hashimoto's (including me) have been amazed at the huge difference that properly digesting food can make.

It should be noted that there are some important restrictions to consider before taking betaine with pepsin:

- Betaine with pepsin should not be used with current ulcers or a history of ulcers, as stomach acid can further aggravate ulcers.
- As NSAIDs and steroid medications can increase the likelihood of developing an ulcer, I do not recommend using this supplement while taking either of these medications. NSAIDs include aspirin, ibuprofen, and naproxen (Bayer, Advil, Aleve, and many others). Steroid medications include prednisone, hydrocortisone, and others.
- Acid-suppressing medications including the popular PPIs mentioned earlier and over-the-counter acid blockers like Pepcid can negate the effects of betaine with pepsin, so I don't recommend taking them together.

If you have Hashimoto's and a history of ulcers, PPI use, NSAID use, or steroid use, I highly recommend testing for gut infections, especially *H. pylori* and SIBO, which could be triggers of gut symptoms and Hashimoto's.

Proteolytic Enzymes

Proteolytic enzymes, also known as systemic enzymes, act as natural immune modulators, meaning they can help bring our immune system into balance. Systemic enzymes are a blend of plant- and animal-derived enzymes and may contain a mix of some of the following ingredients:

- Bromelain (from pineapple)
- Papain (from papaya)
- Rutin or rutoside trihydrate (bioflavonoid)
- Chymotrypsin (porcine)
- Trypsin (porcine)
- Pancreatin (porcine)

Systemic enzymes break down inflammatory cytokines that are seen in autoimmune disease and contain proteases that may also be involved with breaking down pathogens such as bacteria and parasites. These enzymes also speed up tissue repair by reducing inflammation. Additionally, the enzymes reduce the antibodies to foods and to the thyroid by breaking down the CICs that are formed in autoimmune disease.

Systemic enzymes have been studied extensively in Europe and have become a popular alternative to pain medications for arthritic disease and many inflammatory conditions.

A poster presentation at the International Congress on Immuno-rehabilitation Allergy, Immunology, and Global Net in Cannes, France, in 2002 found that Wobenzym, a proprietary blend of systemic enzymes, taken at a dose of five tablets three times per day showed very promising results in Hashimoto's.

In the study, Hashimoto's patients on levothyroxine were given systemic enzymes for three to six months. Not only did patients report a reduction of thyroid symptoms, but thyroid ultrasounds also showed normalization, and there was a reduced number of inflammatory cells in the thyroid and significant decreases in TPO and TG antibodies. Many of these patients were able to reduce their dose of levothyroxine, and some were able to discontinue their medications completely. Cholesterol profiles also improved in the patients who had high cholesterol levels before starting the enzymes.

In my work with Hashimoto's patients, I've seen an equally positive response. Systemic enzyme supplementation for one to three months has shown to help significantly reduce both thyroid antibodies and food sensitivities. An extra bonus is that because systemic enzymes act on the immune system as a whole, using them is considered to be protective against developing future autoimmune conditions.

The key to remember about these enzymes is that they are to be taken *without* food. This means either on an empty stomach, at least forty-five minutes before a meal, or an hour and a half after a meal. If you take them with food or too soon after you've eaten, they will get used up in the process of digestion instead of making their way into the bloodstream, where they can act on CICs.

While most systemic enzyme product labels will state to take six capsules daily, this is typically considered to be more of a maintenance dose. The dose of enzymes used in the Cannes study was 2.5 times higher than this, or five capsules three times per day, taken on an empty stomach, and this is the dose I recommend. Experienced clinicians will use this higher dose and recommend that it be taken with a full glass of water (at least eight ounces). In some cases, even ten capsules three times per day may be used in the acute phase to modulate the immune system effectively.

Step 3: Balance the Gut Flora

Balancing the bacterial flora in the gut can play a critical role in overcoming autoimmune conditions by helping normalize intestinal permeability. When our bacterial flora is not balanced, this contributes to the autoimmune condition through continuous antigen stimulation.

Eating a variety of foods contributes to a healthy gut flora. However, this is often challenging to do in the early phases of healing Hashimoto's. During this time, we need to rely on external sources of beneficial flora, including from fermented foods and probiotic supplements.

Fermented Foods

Fermented foods like sauerkraut and other fermented vegetables (that are kept in the refrigerator section of the grocery store or are homemade and refrigerated) have an abundance of beneficial bacteria and can be very helpful in rebalancing the gut flora. Kefir and yogurt are also filled with good bacteria, but if you are sensitive to dairy proteins, these options won't work for you and you should instead try fermented coconut water or fermented coconut yogurt.

I have found that most people with Hashimoto's can really benefit from fermented foods. However, others, such as those with SIBO, may have an adverse reaction.

Try my Fermented Margarita for inspiration (see page 129).

Probiotics

Probiotics are widely used to rebalance the gut flora. The beneficial bacteria in probiotics should help displace the pathogenic bacteria and reestablish the balance we are seeking. The key with probiotic supplementation is not to overdo it right away but instead to focus on starting small and then gradually increasing the dosage until a die-off reaction is felt. A die-off reaction—also known as a Jarisch-Herxheimer reaction, or sometimes just Herxheimer or Herx—occurs when the dying pathogenic bacteria release endotoxins at a quicker rate than the body can clear them.

Symptoms of a die-off reaction include lethargy, difficulty concentrating, cravings for sweets, diarrhea, rash, irritability, gas, bloating, headache, nausea, vomiting, congestion, and increased autoimmune symptoms. If the die-off reaction is too severe, the dose may be reduced a bit, but it should resolve within three to five days while the probiotic dose is continued. Though the process doesn't sound fun, many people find that they feel significantly better once they endure the short discomfort!

Please note that not all probiotics are created equally. Many drugstore and health food store brands found on the shelves have a very low concentration of probiotic bacteria, which is not enough to correct the gut imbalances in autoimmune disease. I've found three types of probiotics to be helpful for people with Hashimoto's: lactic acid, *Saccharomyces boulardii* (*S. boulardii*), and spore-based probiotics.

Lactobacillus-based—lactic acid—probiotics are the most commonly used and can be very helpful in rebalancing gut dysbiosis. Many people with Hashimoto's test deficient in these probiotic bacteria on stool tests. While I recommend starting low (1 to 10 billion CFUs per day) and increasing slowly, doses of 50 billion to 3,600 billion CFUs per day are needed for therapeutic effect. Oftentimes, the lactic acid probiotics may be mixed in with bifidobacteria-based probiotics and sometimes *Streptococcus* probiotics. I have found that high-dose blends of multiple strains seem to

Probiotic Blends

Probiotic Type	Best Products
Lactic acid based	VSL#3, Ther-Biotic Complete by Klaire Labs, Probiotic 50B by Pure Encapsulations
Yeast based	*Saccharomyces boulardii* by Pure Encapsulations
Spore based	MegaSporeBiotic, Rootcology MegaSpore

do best. *Lactobacillus casei* has specifically been found to aid with healing the gut. *Pediococcus acidilactici* is a lactic acid probiotic that has been found to downregulate autoimmunity by increasing the expression of T-regulatory cells, which help to reduce the inflammatory autoimmune cascade.

These probiotics can be very helpful for people with Hashimoto's who often show low levels of them on gut lab tests. However, they may be problematic for people with SIBO, which can be caused by an overgrowth of various bacteria, including *Lactobacillus* and *Streptococcus* bacteria, which are often found in probiotics. It's important to note that up to 50 percent of people with Hashimoto's may have SIBO, and up to 75 percent may have an overgrowth of *Lactobacillus* or *Streptococcus* bacteria. Please see chapter 11 on infections for more information.

Beneficial yeast-based *S. boulardii* is a beneficial yeast that helps to raise our secretory IgA, which acts as a protective barrier in the gut, leading to a removal of opportunistic and pathogenic organisms from the gut and preventing new infections as well as reinfections. This type of probiotic is an excellent tool for addressing dysbiosis, yeast overgrowth, and parasitic infections, and it can be used concurrently with antibiotics. Furthermore, yeast-based probiotics do not have a propensity to increase SIBO. I recommend a dose of 250 mg to 2,000 mg per day.

Spore-based probiotics just recently came on my radar after some colleagues reported having excellent results with these types of probiotics. Spore-based probiotics are natural and soil-based and have a unique mechanism of action, which allows them to directly modulate the gut microbiome. Spore-based probiotics have shown promise in various autoimmune diseases and in reducing allergies and asthma. Spore-based probiotics also have an ability to boost *Lactobacillus* colonies, so they can be used concurrently with *Lactobacillus* probiotics as well as in place of them. Unlike the *Lactobacillus* probiotics, spore-based probiotics can reduce SIBO and increase gut diversity by boosting the growth of other beneficial flora.

Clients and colleagues with Hashimoto's have reported the following after using for thirty to ninety days: a reduction in thyroid antibodies, an improved mood, less pain, better bowel movements, more energy, and a reduction or complete elimination of food sensitivities.

The starting dose for spore-based probiotics is one capsule every other day, and the therapeutic dose is two capsules per day. Once the desired effect has been seen (generally three to six months in people with Hashimoto's), I recommend dropping down to a maintenance dose of one capsule per day.

Step 4: Nourish the Gut

Easy Bone Broth

5 chicken legs

2 cups mixed chopped carrots, onions, and celery

1 tablespoon apple cider vinegar

Sea salt to taste

Purified water

Add all ingredients to a slow cooker and cook overnight to wake up to delicious bone broth. According to Dr. Kellyann Petrucci, author of *Bone Broth Diet,* bone broth should cook for 8 to 24 hours to extract the most nutrients. Cooking bone broth in a slow cooker is the best way to do so and is so much easier than using a stovetop!

Removing reactive foods and using probiotics and systemic enzymes will go a long way toward gut repair, but completing those three steps alone might leave you without the support you need to sustain long-term gut health. For that, it's recommended that you nourish your gut with bone broth and add in supplemental L-glutamine, zinc, NAC, omega-3 fatty acids, and vitamin D.

Glutamine

Glutamine is the best-studied substance for healing intestinal permeability. Supplementation of this important amino acid has been found to reduce the leaky gut associated with the use of NSAIDs and abdominal surgery. A deficiency in glutamine is also known to cause increased intestinal permeability in mouse models and malnourished children.

New gut cells are produced within the GI tract every three to six days, and glutamine can help repair the GI lining in collaboration with other amino acids such as leucine and arginine. The recommended adult dose is 5 g three times per day; however, higher doses have been used.

Zinc

Zinc is an essential element for our well-being. Zinc acts as a catalyst in about a hundred different enzyme reactions that take place within the body, and it is involved in DNA synthesis, immune function, protein synthesis, and cell division. It is required for proper sense of taste and smell, detoxification, wound healing, and thyroid function.

One in four individuals in the general population may be zinc deficient, including most people with hypothyroidism. Zinc deficiency prevents the conversion of T4 into the active T3 version. You also need zinc to form TSH, which is why people who are constantly producing TSH—those with hypothyroidism—are more likely to develop deficiencies in this important mineral.

If you have celiac disease or any other malabsorption syndrome that has caused intestinal damage, you may have an impaired ability to absorb zinc. Poor zinc absorption can also be caused by eating phytate-containing foods such as grains, legumes, nuts, and seeds with zinc-containing foods, or taking iron supplements with meals (iron can interfere with the absorption of zinc from foods).

Zinc plays a specific role in gut health, as deficiency has been associated with increased intestinal permeability, susceptibility to infections, and reduced detoxification of bacterial toxins. In conditions such as Crohn's disease, replenishing zinc has shown to help repair intestinal permeability.

Because zinc is not stored in the body, a daily intake is recommended even for the general population, and people with Hashimoto's and other autoimmune conditions should consider zinc supplementation a part of their everyday regimen.

Symptoms of zinc deficiency can include poor wound healing, impaired taste and smell, and thin, brittle, peeling, or white-spotted nails. Tests such as the SpectraCell Laboratories micronutrient test will show your zinc levels, although a deficiency can also be detected in a liver function blood test, where it will present as low alkaline phosphatase levels.

In order to address deficiency, zinc supplementation can be used, but doses should be no more than 30 mg per day without doctor's supervision. Doses above 40 mg may cause a depletion in copper levels. In research, 50 mg of zinc taken over ten weeks led to depletions in both copper and iron. In some cases, like when we're copper toxic, that's a good thing. In others, it can produce a copper deficiency, and you may need to take supplemental copper. Symptoms of copper deficiency are anemia not responsive to iron supplements, trouble with walking and balance, fatigue, and light-headedness.

You can also look to add zinc through diet. Oysters have the highest concentration of zinc, but they are not typically considered an everyday food. Beef, liver, pork, lobster, and chicken are the next best sources of zinc. It is easier to extract zinc from meat than nonmeat sources, which is why vegetarians will have an increased risk of zinc deficiency.

Not all supplemental zinc formulations are created equally. I prefer the zinc picolinate version because it is absorbed better. To ensure optimal absorption, zinc supplements should be taken with food.

NAC

I consider N-acetylcysteine (NAC) to be a super supplement for people with Hashimoto's. NAC turns into glutathione in the body and not only supports liver function but also helps to clear out heavy metals and promotes intestinal health by helping to detoxify intestinal bacteria and by breaking down biofilms that house gut pathogens. Hashimoto's patients are often deficient in the antioxidant glutathione, which helps prevent free radical damage to the thyroid. NAC has been used for healing intestinal permeability and should be taken orally. It's important to note that it can cause stomach upset if taken on an empty stomach and should be taken with food. If you followed the Liver Support Protocol, you should have already started taking NAC, and I recommend that you continue taking it for three to six months.

Omega-3 Fatty Acids

Omega-3 fatty acids can help reduce inflammation and are found primarily in fish, shellfish, and flaxseeds, although they can also be taken in supplement form for those who cannot eat adequate amounts of fish or are concerned about mercury content.

Our immune functions work best when we have enough omega-3 and omega-6 fats, ideally at a 1:1 ratio. The problem is most people get too many omega-6 fatty acids, which are found in vegetable oils such as canola, corn, soybean, peanut, sunflower, safflower, cottonseed, and grapeseed, and in margarine and shortening. You consume these fats when you eat processed salad dressings, store-bought condiments, chips, artificial cheeses, store-bought roasted nuts, cookies, crackers, snack foods, sauces, and almost everything in the middle aisles of the grocery store.

Since omega-6 fats can promote inflammation, you'll want to minimize their intake and instead focus on consuming more omega-3 fats. Look to fish and flaxseed products and to high-quality supplements. Omega-3 acid supplementation has been found to be helpful in a variety of autoimmune conditions and has the power to reduce inflammation. Doses of 1 to 4 g are recommended.

Vitamin D

Vitamin D deficiency is more commonly found in people with Hashimoto's—68 percent of my readers with Hashimoto's reported also being diagnosed with vitamin D deficiency—and deficiency has been correlated with the presence of antithyroid antibodies. Research done in Turkey found that 92 percent of Hashimoto's patients were deficient in vitamin D, and another 2013 study found that low vitamin D levels were associated with higher thyroid antibodies and worse disease prognosis.

Vitamin D plays an important role in immune balance, building resiliency against infections like the Epstein-Barr virus and in maintaining gut health. Scientists believe that autoimmune conditions are more likely to cluster in regions farther from the equator because of inadequate vitamin D levels—vitamin D is primarily absorbed via sunshine on skin that is free of sunscreen.

Vitamin D is shown to prevent and modulate autoimmunity, and I believe it is especially important for people who have had a prior Epstein-Barr infection (this infection can often trigger Hashimoto's and create a chronic low-grade infection), as the cells that fight the virus (CD8+ T cells) are vitamin D dependent.

Vitamin D has been helpful in my recovery, and I've found that exposure to sunshine is consistently something that makes my clients and readers feel better. Furthermore, a sampling of clients who reported feeling well or being in remission showed that most of them had their vitamin D levels in the optimal range.

A recommended daily allowance of 400 IU has been established, but studies are showing this is not adequate for most people. I generally recommend 5,000 IU per day as a starting point for my clients with Hashimoto's. However, I also recommend monitoring vitamin D levels to ensure that the person is within the optimal range (60 to 80 ng/mL for optimal thyroid receptor and immune system function). In some cases, practitioners may utilize doses as high as 20,000 IU to get to the goal, but I would not recommend doing this on your own, as vitamin D can build up.

Your Prescription? A Beach Vacation!

The best way to restore optimal vitamin D level is through sun exposure, safe tanning beds, and an oral vitamin D_3 supplement. The secondary best sources of vitamin D are from foods like wild salmon (800 IU of D_3 per 3.5 ounces of salmon) and cod liver oil (700 IU per teaspoon). However, people with fat malabsorption may not properly absorb vitamin D from foods.

Vitamin D advocates recommend fifteen minutes of sun on exposed skin without sunscreen around noon. Perhaps you can go for a walk during lunchtime. If you are fair skinned and not used to the sun, you may not be able to tolerate so much sun exposure at first and may need to experience it gradually while taking a vitamin D supplement. Be careful not to overexpose yourself to prevent getting sunburned.

However, some health care professionals suggested that in severe deficiency, getting adequate vitamin D levels would require you to spend four to six hours exposed on a sunny beach for seven days straight! Unless you have a beach vacation planned (bring me?), taking a vitamin D_3 supplement is your best bet.

GUT BALANCE SUPPLEMENTS

Systemic enzymes (see recommended brands): 10 capsules or tablets, 3 times per day on an empty stomach

Probiotics: Work your way up to target dose

L-glutamine powder: 5 g, 3 times per day

Zinc: 30 mg per day

NAC: 1,800 mg per day

Omega-3s: 1–4 g per day

Vitamin D: 5,000 IU per day

The Gut Balance Protocol will help you overcome dysbiosis and some gut infections, but if you find that you still have gut symptoms after completing this protocol, I recommend that you do further investigation through the Advanced Protocols. You may find that you have gut infections and other triggers that require further intervention. Continue this Fundamental Gut Balance Protocol during your infection-eradication phase and for three to six months after to help further seal and heal the gut.

Next Steps and Roadblocks

After you've completed the Fundamental Protocols, be sure to take the Thyroid Symptom Assessment from page 62 again. What changes and improvements did you notice?

Fundamental Tests: Ferritin, Vitamin D, and B₁₂

Many people who are diagnosed with Hashimoto's will present with low levels of vitamin D, vitamin B_{12}, and ferritin, the iron storage protein. Eating a nutrient-dense diet that is free of reactive foods will usually help with many of these deficiencies. However, supplementation may be necessary in many cases, especially in the event of long-standing, severe, and multiple-nutrient deficiency.

I recommend that you ask your doctor to order tests for ferritin, vitamin D, and vitamin B_{12} and then supplement accordingly based on your results. For vitamin D, there are two available tests: 1,25 (OH)D and 25(OH)D. The test 25(OH)D, also called 25-hydroxy vitamin D, is preferred. Furthermore, these nutrients should be monitored every three to six months when supplementing to ensure that you are getting adequate and not excessive amounts. Please see chapter 9 for more information on interpreting labs and supplementing correctly. These tests should be covered by most insurance companies, but if your doctor will not order the tests for you or you have a high deductible, you can self-order them. Please see the action plan at www.thyroidpharmacist.com/action for more information.

If you're like 80 percent of the clients I've worked with over the last few years, you are feeling significantly better after completing the Fundamental Protocols. If, however, you are still feeling less than 100 percent after you've completed the Liver Support, Adrenal Recovery, and Gut Balance Protocols, or if you continue to have elevated thyroid antibodies, I recommend you dig deeper to specific root causes and triggers that may be contributing to your symptoms and the condition. This is why I designed the book this way with Fundamental and Advanced Protocols. The goal is to help everyone reverse symptoms and get back to feeling healthy again. Turn the page to find the tools you need to dig further.

GUT-HEALTH SUPPLEMENT OVERVIEW

Supplement Type	Action	Recommended Brand	Notes
Betaine with pepsin	Helps digest protein-containing meals	Pure Encapsulations	Take with protein-containing meals. Do not use with ulcers, *H. pylori*, NSAIDs, steroids, or proton pump inhibitors, or if burning occurs after taking.
Systemic and proteolytic enzymes	Break down circulating immune complexes, antibodies to the thyroid gland, and foods	Wobenzym PS, Pure Encapsulations Systemic Enzyme Complex	May impact clotting tests. Stop for 2 weeks prior to any surgery.
Probiotic	Works to balance beneficial flora	Rootcology, MegaSporeBiotic, Klaire Labs, VSL#3, Pure Encapsulations	Do not take *lactobacillus*-containing probiotics with SIBO.
L-glutamine powder	5 g, 3 times per day helps to repair leaky gut	Pure Encapsulations	Do not take if feeling too agitated.

Supplement Type	Action	Recommended Brand	Notes
Zinc picolinate	30 mg daily helps to support the gut barrier	Pure Encapsulations	Take with food. May deplete iron, copper.
N-acetylcysteine (NAC)	Supports liver function, breaks down pathogenic biofilms in the gut, supports glutathione levels	Pure Encapsulations, Rootcology	Take with food. May cause discomfort on empty stomach.
Omega-3 fatty acids	1–4 g reduces inflammation and heals the gut	Pure Encapsulations EPA/DHA	If burping occurs after taking, freeze before taking.
Vitamin D	Supports immune function and gut integrity	Pure Encapsulations	Start with 5,000 IU per day, then adjust based on lab values. May build up in the body, so test within 3–6 months of starting supplement.

THE FULL FUNDAMENTAL PROTOCOLS

Here's an overview of the complete Fundamental Protocols and the steps of each individual protocol contained within.

Focus and Length	Overview
Liver (2 weeks)	Overview: Remove potentially triggering foods, add supportive foods, reduce toxic exposure, support detox pathways
	Diet: Root Cause Intro diet: remove gluten, dairy, soy, sugar
	Supplements: Liver reset powder, NAC, methylation support, magnesium
	Benefits: Eliminate overall toxic exposure, improve body's detoxification abilities, reduce body's toxic burden
Adrenal (4 weeks)	Overview: Rest, de-stress, reduce inflammation, balance the blood sugar, replenish nutrients and add adaptogens
	Diet: Root Cause Paleo Diet: remove grains
	Supplements: Adrenal adaptogens, B vitamins, magnesium, selenium, thiamine, vitamin C
	Benefits: Shift body into a regenerative process, increase strength and resilience, rebalance inflammatory hormones
Gut (6 weeks)	Overview: Remove reactive foods, supplement with enzymes, balance the gut flora, nourish the gut
	Diet: Root Cause Autoimmune Diet: remove gut-reactive foods including eggs, nightshades, seeds, nuts

Focus and Length	Overview
Gut (continued)	Supplements: Betaine, L-glutamine, omega-3 probiotics, systemic enzymes, vitamin D, zinc
	Benefits: Renew bacterial and microbial balance, eliminate digestive distress, reduce autoimmune expression

7

Advanced Root Cause Assessments

f you've reached this point in the book, you are familiar with the Fundamental Protocols, which will help correct your underlying vulnerabilities. In a large number of people, completing the Fundamental Protocols alone results in a significant improvement in their Hashimoto's-related symptoms. Yet if you've worked through these protocols and still don't feel quite like yourself, don't worry—help is here! I'm going to guide you through a deeper investigation that will help prioritize the next steps for your treatment.

This investigation will include taking a closer look at your own personal health timeline and seeing where we might identify risk factors you might have had before developing Hashimoto's. You will need to think as far back as you can remember to establish your overall health history and make note of underlying events or triggers that could have contributed to your illness. Once identified, these triggers will have to be addressed before you can achieve complete wellness.

I've designed a series of assessments that will help identify your personal triggers and prioritize the next steps of your unique protocol. There are more than twenty potential triggers, and going through medical testing for them all without a clear sense of direction can become overwhelming and expensive. Rather than traveling down that indirect and frustrating path, I recommend that you complete the assessments in this chapter and let your scores reveal which of the Advanced Protocols should be a priority.

Before doing so, however, let's first define what a trigger is in the context of autoimmunity and specifically in Hashimoto's.

Defining Triggers and Their Role in the Advanced Protocols

I like to think of triggers in terms of antigenic load. An antigen is a substance that causes the immune system to make antibodies against it and can be a chemical, bacterium, virus, or pollen particle, as well as a toxin or cell. When there are too many antigens in the body, the immune system can become overwhelmed and lose its ability to distinguish self from non-self. When the immune system attacks the self—or the body instead of the antigens—this is autoimmune disease.

In my work, I've found that there is often a combination of antigens that act as a trigger for Hashimoto's, and that a trigger can be anything that has the potential to stress the body or mind, upset the gut barrier, or clog up our detox pathways. Well-established environmental triggers for developing Hashimoto's in those who are genetically predisposed include excessive iodine intake, selenium deficiency, hormonal imbalances, toxins, and therapy with certain types of medications. Scientific studies have also correlated Hashimoto's onset with the hormonal shifts that occur with pregnancy, puberty, and perimenopause.

From an adaptive physiology standpoint, a trigger is anything that can make our body think that it's best to conserve, rather than expend, energy.

To create your personal health timeline, it's important to consider all potential Hashimoto's triggers to which you may have been exposed. When you look at this list of potential triggers, do you see any you've personally encountered or experienced?

☐ Accutane (acne medication)
☐ Amiodarone (heart medication)
☐ Bacterial infection
☐ Blood transfusion
☐ Cytomegalovirus
☐ Dental x-rays
☐ Emotional stress
☐ Epstein-Barr virus
☐ Excessive iodine intake
☐ Fluoride exposure
☐ Heavy metals
☐ *H. pylori* bacteria
☐ Hepatitis C virus
☐ Hepatitis C treatment
☐ Herpes virus
☐ HPV vaccine
☐ Interferon- and cytokine-based medications

☐ Lithium (medication used for bipolar disorder)
☐ Lyme disease or tick bites
☐ Mold
☐ Parasites
☐ Periodontal pathogens
☐ Pregnancy
☐ Radiation
☐ Selenium deficiency
☐ Stress
☐ Toxin exposure
☐ Trauma to the neck
☐ Tyrosine kinase inhibitors (medications used for cancer)
☐ Viral infection
☐ Whiplash
☐ *Yersinia* bacteria

Once you've identified your triggers, the next step is to address them head-on to help ensure optimum healing. In the Advanced Protocols, you will find a chapter on the ever-important art of optimizing thyroid hormone levels using medications, innovative technologies, and natural means. After that, I've organized the four most common categories of triggers: foods, stress, infections, and toxins. Each of these categories will get its very own chapter and specific protocol. Which specific protocol you should start with will depend on your scores when you complete the Advanced Root Cause Assessments.

The Root Cause Assessments

Hashimoto's results when our body receives a message to self-destruct based on the signals in our environment. Factors like nutrient depletions, food sensitivities, toxins, stress, intestinal permeability, and infections are root causes that result in thyroid hormone abnormalities.

In rare cases, a person may have just one root cause, but in most cases, a person will have multiple root causes. Thus a comprehensive approach will be needed to recover.

In the Fundamental Protocols, we addressed multiple nutrient deficiencies, food sensitivities, and gut imbalances; helped your body clear out toxins; and boosted your body's resilience to stress. These strategies will help you feel better, no matter your root cause. The Advanced Protocols will help you uncover additional triggers. You will see improvement in your health with each trigger you address!

You have two ways to approach the Advanced Protocols:

- You can do the Fundamental Protocols first and then follow up with the assessments if you are still having symptoms or immune imbalance. These will help you do some digging into your specific root causes and imbalances.
- You can do the following assessments and related Advanced Protocols as you go through the Fundamental Protocols to help you recover faster.

Please go through the following assessments and mark the statements that apply to you. If you have one or more symptoms on an assessment, this is an indication that you need to do further testing and digging within the related Advanced Protocol.

THYROID HORMONES ASSESSMENT
Mark which symptoms apply to you.

- ☐ I have tangled, thinning hair or hair loss.
- ☐ My eyebrows are thinning.
- ☐ My face looks puffy.
- ☐ I experience memory loss or brain fog.
- ☐ I experience sadness or apathy.

☐ I am fatigued.
☐ I hardly ever sweat.
☐ I'm colder than the average person.
☐ I have gained weight and have trouble losing weight.
☐ I experience joint pain.
☐ I tend to have heavy menstrual periods.
☐ I feel irritable, agitated, or restless and have mood swings.
☐ I have palpitations or a rapid heart rate.
☐ I can't stand the heat.
☐ My periods have been scanty or light.
☐ I am experiencing unintentional weight loss.
☐ I struggle with insomnia.
☐ I am sweating excessively.

Thyroid hormone assessment score: ____

NUTRITION ASSESSMENT

Mark which symptoms apply to you.

☐ I was a vegetarian for more than six months.
☐ I was a vegan for more than three months.
☐ I eat processed or packaged foods.
☐ I have never had a nutritional consult.
☐ My wounds heal slowly.
☐ I have been anemic before.
☐ I eat a low-fat diet.
☐ I have multiple strange symptoms.
☐ I don't tan well and don't spend at least two hours in the sun each day.
☐ I have dry skin, dandruff, or dry hair.
☐ I eat fewer than six servings of vegetables per day.
☐ I have multiple food sensitivities.
☐ My diet is very restricted.
☐ I have a history of an eating disorder like anorexia, bulimia, binge eating, or orthorexia.
☐ I have never had food sensitivity testing.
☐ I have multiple autoimmune conditions.

Nutrition assessment score: ____

TRAUMATIC STRESS ASSESSMENT

Mark which symptoms apply to you.

☐ I experienced a premature loss of a loved one.

☐ I had an abusive or traumatic childhood.

☐ I have felt socially isolated during my life.

☐ I have been in an abusive relationship.

☐ I am not in a happy or fulfilling relationship.

☐ I worry a lot or feel the world is an unsafe place.

☐ I overcommit and have a hard time saying no.

☐ I feel guilty or ashamed more than once a year.

☐ I don't have friends I can trust.

☐ I feel frustrated often, am quick to get angry, or am slow to forgive or get over things.

☐ I often play the role of the martyr or feel like others are taking advantage of me.

☐ I am always tired. Everyday tasks are an effort, and stress feels overwhelming.

☐ I tend to be a night owl, or I have a hard time waking up in the morning.

☐ I sleep too much or not enough, or I don't feel rested after sleeping.

☐ I have a hard time expressing myself and speaking up in groups, or I tend to be shy.

☐ I don't have time to play, or I don't have a creative outlet or stress-reducing hobbies.

☐ I have low blood pressure or feel light-headed when I get up too quickly.

☐ I have PMS, irregular periods, infertility, or decreased sex drive.

☐ I have intense cravings for salty foods (aka "I just ate a whole bag of chips" syndrome).

☐ It takes me a long time to recover from illness, my wounds heal slowly, and exercise and stress can leave me exhausted for days.

Traumatic stress assessment score: ____

INFECTIONS ASSESSMENT

Mark which symptoms apply to you.

☐ I had a mystery illness and have never felt the same after.

☐ I have had Epstein-Barr virus (mono), herpes virus, or cytomegalovirus.

☐ I have nasal congestion or sinusitis.

☐ I have swollen lymph glands or a sore throat.

☐ I have a chronic, low-grade fever.

☐ I have irritable bowel syndrome.

☐ I have acid reflux.

☐ I have food sensitivities to more than one food.

☐ I have foul-smelling stools, diarrhea, or flatulence.

☐ I am deficient in ferritin, iron, or B_{12}.

☐ I have experienced food poisoning.

☐ I crave alcohol or sweets.

☐ My gums bleed when I brush my teeth.

☐ I have dental pain, receding gums, or bad breath.

☐ I have constipation, diarrhea, bloating, indigestion, malabsorption, or stomach cramps more than once per month.

☐ I have been camping, have been bitten by a tick, or live in a Lyme-endemic area.

☐ I have pain anywhere in my body.

☐ I have hives, rashes, allergies, or asthma.

Infections assessment score: ___

TOXINS ASSESSMENT

Mark which symptoms apply to you.

☐ I have skin rashes, breakouts, and other types of skin reactions.

☐ I have multiple chemical or odor sensitivities.

☐ I have or have had dental amalgams (silver fillings).

☐ I have consumed tuna more than twenty times per year.

☐ I have fatigue that is not caused by obvious reasons like exercise or staying up late.

☐ I do not tolerate alcohol.

☐ I've had significant exposure to chemicals like pesticides, cosmetics, plastics, or industrial chemicals.

☐ I've lived in a place with mold.

☐ I have taken oral contraceptives for more than one year.

☐ I have a history of blood clots in my body or menstrual cycle.

☐ I have worked on a farm, in a dental office, in a factory, or as a painter.

☐ I've lived in a big metropolitan city for over one year.

☐ I hardly sweat.
☐ I have the MTHFR gene mutation.
☐ I have a family history of birth defects.
☐ I have sinusitis.
☐ I was a vegetarian for more than three months.
☐ I have tingling in my extremities.
☐ I have a rapid pulse.
☐ I have a metallic taste in my mouth.

Toxins assessment score: ___

Now that you've identified your potential root causes, it's time to start addressing them!

PART III

THE ADVANCED
PROTOCOLS

8

Protocols for Optimizing
Thyroid Hormones

I f you're like most people with Hashimoto's, you will benefit from optimizing your thyroid hormone levels. In this chapter, I'll discuss five unique strategies that will assist with optimizing your thyroid hormone levels: prescription thyroid hormones, the immune-modulating medication low-dose naltrexone, low-level laser therapy, glandulars, and some complementary aromatherapy protocols.

Before we jump into the first strategy of prescription hormones, I want to address goal setting as it relates to thyroid medications. This is a topic that comes up with some of my clients who first come to work with me and state that they'd like to prevent having to take medications or that they are looking to reduce their dependency on thyroid medications. I explain to them that while I think this may be a reasonable long-term goal, for some people we need to use thyroid medications to optimize hormone levels in the short term. Thyroid hormone receptors are present in just about every cell in the body and have the important role of controlling numerous body functions including our metabolism (which is crucial to healing). If thyroid hormone levels aren't properly supported, you risk delaying and even sabotaging your own recovery.

Prescription Thyroid Hormones

Getting on replacement thyroid hormone medications is an important step to feeling well with Hashimoto's. When used appropriately, medications are the quickest and most effective way to reduce thyroid symptoms, limit the autoimmune attack on the thyroid gland, shrink goiter size, lessen the likelihood of thyroid cancer, and give you the energy and clarity of mind to keep working toward improving your health.

Thyroid medications can be of tremendous benefit while we fix the issues contributing to our autoimmune thyroiditis. We know that Hashimoto's is a progressive condition, and in many cases, significant damage has occurred to the thyroid gland, so medications are a must. As a pharmacist, I recognize that medications are a great tool in helping people overcome Hashimoto's, but as my protocols suggest, they shouldn't be considered the only part of your arsenal.

If you're not yet taking thyroid medications, this section will help you determine whether they would be appropriate for you. If you're already taking thyroid medications, you may be surprised to learn that you may not be getting the optimal treatment, and you'll discover the tools needed to optimize your medications while working with your physician. Getting on the right kind of thyroid medication at the right dose and taking it in the right way can make a tremendous difference in your symptoms, especially in energy, weight, brain function, and hair appearance.

The Four Rs of Optimal Thyroid Medication Use

I'm going to share the four most common medication-related considerations that thyroid patients and their health care team need to make. These are the four Rs of optimal thyroid medication use, and they include guidance for various scenarios to help ensure you find the right balance for thyroid medication.

1. Right Person: Are You a Candidate for Thyroid Medications?

Are you a candidate for thyroid medications? This is an important question to address, as I oftentimes see people who should be on thyroid medications who are refused treatment *by* their doctors (and sometimes the patients themselves refuse treatments *from* their doctors). If you have an elevation of TSH above 2.0 µIU/mL, thyroid symptoms, or thyroid antibodies, there is a likely chance that thyroid medications will help you.

Researchers have found that taking external thyroid hormones results in reduced inflammation in the thyroid, reduced thyroid antibodies, fewer thyroid symptoms, and a slowing of the progression of the condition. This is because external hormones allow our own thyroid gland to turn down internal hormone production, which reduces the overall oxidative stress that is partially generated when an underactive thyroid works hard to produce thyroid hormones.

If your TSH is elevated for a prolonged period of time, not taking thyroid hormones can actually be harmful and may be hindering your recovery. Some people are averse to taking any foreign substance. However, as a pharmacist, I can tell you that thyroid medications are not a foreign substance—they are bioidentical to our internally produced hormones. While some medications cause significant side effects because of how they artificially manipulate our body's chemical messengers, most side effects from thyroid medications are actually due to improper dosing of thyroid hormones. Do not think of medications as a life sentence. Think of them as a helpful tool to get you feeling better. In some cases, you may be able to get off them once you fix the "leaks" in your body that are contributing to the autoimmune destruction of the thyroid.

If you have elevated thyroid antibodies, an elevated TSH, or thyroid symptoms, you may want to talk to your doctor about thyroid hormones. There is no need to suffer while you search for the root cause of your condition.

If you have Addison's disease, cardiovascular disease, or diabetes, thyroid medications should be used with caution, as they may exacerbate the symptoms of these conditions. I also recommend caution if you take amphetamine or stimulant medications, which can interact with thyroid hormones. If you are currently taking any medications, please check with your doctor or pharmacist to discuss potential drug interaction.

2. Right Way: Are You Taking Your Medications to Ensure Proper Absorption?

I often see that patients are not properly counseled about ensuring thyroid medication absorption, which results in them not taking their medications correctly. Many of the strategies in this section will depend on collaboration between you and your doctor. However, you can take full charge of taking your thyroid medication correctly to ensure that you properly absorb the medications.

Absorption of thyroid hormones occurs in the duodenum and jejunum of the small intestine and can be impaired by foods, beverages, medications, supplements, internal factors, and more. I suspect an absorption issue in people who need high doses of thyroid medications or in those who have inconsistent results on thyroid labs despite taking the same dose of medications.

Here are some factors that may impair proper thyroid hormone absorption:

- Stomach acid
- Drug interactions
- Food
- Coffee
- Gut disorders

Let's look at each of these in more detail.

Absorption of thyroid hormones requires the presence of stomach acid, which is why impaired absorption may be seen in patients with low levels of stomach acid (hypochlorhydria) and in those who do not make any stomach acid (achlorhydria).

Some of my clients and readers with low stomach acid have found that taking thyroid medications with hot lemon water (the juice of one lemon in an eight-ounce glass of water) or with apple cider vinegar (one teaspoon per eight-ounce glass of water) can help provide enough acidity to aid with the absorption of thyroid hormones. (The Fundamental Gut Balance Protocol and the Advanced Protocols for addressing infections dive deeper into root causes of low stomach acid.)

Drug interactions also have an effect on thyroid hormone absorption. Antacids, proton pump inhibitors (PPIs), calcium, magnesium, aluminum, and iron can also suppress stomach acid, leading to impaired absorption of thyroid hormones. I always recommend spacing these out from thyroid medications by at least four hours. Most other supplements and medications should be taken thirty to sixty minutes after thyroid medications.

If you are currently taking acid-suppressing medications for acid reflux, I suggest that a careful reevaluation of these meds be done with your doctor. Acid-suppressing medications can exacerbate low stomach acid, which is again common in Hashimoto's and has symptoms identical to those seen in acid reflux. If you are taking any type of PPI medication, please note that these need to be tapered to prevent rebound symptoms.

Food can impair the absorption of thyroid hormones, which is why I always recommend taking thyroid hormones on an empty stomach. A person with normal digestive function can take thyroid medications fifteen to thirty minutes prior to breakfast and have the medications be well absorbed, but some people may need to postpone breakfast by a minimum of sixty minutes after taking thyroid medications for proper absorption. One study found that some people had to wait as long as five hours to eat breakfast to properly absorb their thyroid medications. If you find that your thyroid labs are all over the place or that you need increasingly higher doses of medications, this could be an indication that you need a longer time between your medications and eating.

I recommend keeping thyroid medications at your bedside (keep out of reach of children and pets!) and taking them as soon as you wake up and then waiting at least thirty minutes before eating. Alternative dosing strategies like bedtime dosing or twice per day (usually morning and afternoon) may be used as well and can work better for some people. In this case, taking the medications one hour before eating or two hours after eating is recommended.

Having coffee with thyroid medications can significantly alter, even prevent, the absorption of thyroid medications. Italian researchers found that their espresso-loving patients did not absorb thyroid medications correctly. One person who had an espresso within ten minutes of thyroid medications had a consistently elevated TSH between 13 µIU/mL and 18 µIU/mL. When the same person on the same dose of medication was instructed to take her medication with a full glass of water and then wait one hour to have her coffee, her TSH was testing between to 0.03 and 0.1 µIU/mL for fifteen months! This is why for most patients I recommend waiting thirty to sixty minutes after taking thyroid medications to drink coffee.

Interestingly, a different group of Italian researchers found one specially formulated thyroid medication, called Tirosint, that may withstand the effects of coffee. Tirosint is a gelcap formulation of levothyroxine that showed adequate absorption even when taken with PPIs and coffee. Thank goodness for the research of espresso-loving Italians, right?!

Finally, gut problems, including celiac disease, lactose intolerance, atrophic gastritis, inflammatory bowel disease, and infections like *H. pylori* or parasites can interfere with absorption of thyroid medications. Hopefully, the nutrition changes you've made have helped you absorb your medications and eliminated your gut symptoms. If you still have symptoms such as food intolerance, irritable bowel, or elevated thyroid antibodies after completing the Fundamental Protocols, you likely have a gut infection; please refer to chapter 11 for further guidance.

3. Right Drug: Are You on the Right Type of Medication?

I often see patients taking medications that are not working with their bodies, producing suboptimal results. Synthetic thyroid hormone, commonly known as levothyroxine, is the most commonly utilized thyroid medication. But this is certainly not the only type of thyroid medication that is available. There are three types of medications that can be used to treat an underactive thyroid:

- **Levothyroxine:** This is a T4-containing medication that includes brand names like Synthroid, Levoxyl, Tirosint, Euthyrox (in EU), Eltroxin (in Canada), and Oroxine or Eutroxsig (in Australia). These contain the less-active but longer-acting T4 hormone. The T4 molecule is considered a pro-hormone, as it needs to be converted into the more physiologically active T3 thyroid hormone. T3 is sometimes called our "go" hormone because it tells our body to boost metabolism, grow hair, and create more energy. The conversion from T4 to T3 can be impeded by numerous factors, including stress, nutrient deficiencies, and impaired liver and gut activity.
- **Liothyronine:** T3 medications contain liothyronine and include the brand name Cytomel and compounded T3. These offer the active albeit short-acting T3 hormone. These medications are generally not recommended to be used as a sole therapy for hypothyroidism, as their short half-life may put a person on a thyroid hormone roller coaster. However, they can be used as an add-on to T4-only medications.
- **T4/T3 combination medications:** T4/T3 combination medications offer the two main thyroid hormones in the same ratio that is present in our own bodies. Armour Thyroid, Nature-Throid, and WP Thyroid are known as natural desiccated thyroid (NDT, sometimes called desiccated thyroid extract, or DTE) hormones and are derived from the thyroid glands of pigs. NDT medications also contain the thyroid hormones T1 and T2, which may have some physiological activity as well. Compounded versions of T4/T3 are also available.

It's not by chance that I've had you reduce your stress, address nutrient depletions, and support your gut and liver function before having the medication conversation. All of the actions you've taken to support your body should have improved your conversion from T4 to T3, but if you continue to feel unwell and have hypothyroid symptoms despite already taking a T4-containing medication, you may want to talk to your doctor about switching over to a medication that has preconverted T3 already in the formulation.

Dutch endocrinologist and top thyroid researcher Dr. Wilmar Wiersinga suggests that some people may be genetically unable to properly activate and transport thyroid hormones and may benefit from combination T4/T3 therapy, and that people who continue to have thyroid symptoms despite normal TSH levels may benefit from the addition of T3 into their medication regimen (whether through adding T3 to T4, or by taking a T4/T3 combination medication).

While T4-only and T3-only medications have their place, I've found that most of my clients feel best on combination medications that contain both T4 and T3, such as WP Thyroid, Nature-Throid, Armour Thyroid, compounded T4/T3, or a combination of levothyroxine and liothyronine. Of course, my experience tends to be a biased one, as most of the people who reach out to me are usually not doing well on T4-only medication and are seeking more help with their thyroid. Those who are doing well on T4 alone are not as likely to seek my help!

Another thing to consider when taking thyroid medications is reactions to fillers like corn (in Armour Thyroid), gluten cross-contamination (in Cytomel), lactose (in most thyroid medications except Tirosint and compounded medications), or other ingredients. Top hypoallergenic choices are Tirosint, WP Thyroid, and compounded T4/T3 medications.

Switching between brands of thyroid medications, though sometimes necessary, can mean that a person who was previously

Root Cause Research Corner: Survey Says ...

A survey of over two thousand Root Cause readers revealed the following results regarding which medications made them feel better or worse.

Please use these results to guide your treatment plan, but also remember that you are an individual and not a statistic. Just because most people felt better on a particular medication doesn't mean that this will be your ideal medication.

ROOT CAUSE MEDICATION SURVEY

Medication	Percentage Reported Feeling Better	Percentage Reported Feeling Worse	Percentage No Difference
Armour Thyroid	59	18.5	22.5
Nature-Throid	56.5	11	32.5
Compounded T4/T3	55	11.5	33.5
Cytomel	52	12	36
Synthroid	43	31	26
Tirosint	26	8	66
Levoxyl	25	25	50

stable on a particular dose of medication may require a higher or lower dose of the new brand. Retest your thyroid four to six weeks after switching medications or doses to be sure you are dosed appropriately.

Also, I'd like to caution you about online medications. I strongly suggest you avoid ordering meds online, as these can be counterfeit and unsafe. Medications are medications, and they require that someone is monitoring your lab tests!

The bottom line is that there are many options for thyroid hormone treatment. Each person should work with an open-minded physician to find the thyroid medication that works best for them. Thyroid hormone therapy should be individualized with the patient in mind.

A Peek into Medication Bias

I'll be honest with you—not many conventionally trained doctors and even endocrinologists are going to be willing to prescribe a T3-containing medication. Although research shows that patients prefer T3-containing medications and oftentimes see improved symptoms—like better mood, more energy, increased hair growth, and weight loss—the truth is, T3-containing medications, and especially NDT medications, have a long and complicated history.

In years past, T3 medications were combined with amphetamines and given to overweight people without thyroid disease to produce rapid and dangerous weight loss. Many of today's practicing doctors saw this dangerous practice firsthand and have been apprehensive about using these drugs ever since. NDT medications, on the other hand, have been shown to have dosage discrepancies within batches. These discrepancies were a result of the manufacturer measuring the thyroid medications by the content of iodine (which varied and was not necessarily related to the dose of the drug). However, current NDT manufacturers now use the actual amounts of T4 and T3 to standardize the doses. RLC Labs, the manufacturer of Nature-Throid and WP Thyroid, assert on their website that Nature-Throid has never been recalled for inconsistent T4 and T3 hormones.

Another factor to be considered in conventional doctors' reluctance in switching medications is the influence of pharmaceutical companies. As a former pharmaceutical sales rep, I can tell you that drug companies use their marketing dollars wisely to influence the prescribing habits of doctors. While the industry is much more regulated now, in the past, most medical education was coming directly from pharmaceutical companies with a vested interest in promoting their products. As T3 and NDT medications have long been off patent while Synthroid held an exclusive bioequivalence status for many years, most doctors were directly or indirectly educated about thyroid medication use through the manufacturers of levothyroxine medications. I personally learned that Synthroid was the standard of care in pharmacy school and that NTDs were not reliable. I myself was uncomfortable with T3-containing medications when I graduated from pharmacy school, and most doctors are uncomfortable prescribing something that is outside the standard of care.

One can certainly understand a doctor's aversion to T3 or T4/T3 combinations because of the history of inappropriate use, unstable dosing, and biased education they've received. Most doctors really care about your safety and want to do the best by their patients. And to be fair, you shouldn't ask or expect your doctors to do something they are not comfortable with or experienced in doing. This is why your best bet is to work with a doctor who already knows how to use T3-containing medications safely and effectively. As a patient, you have the right to seek different opinions.

Because each thyroid hormone formulation is dosed differently, I've created a thyroid hormone conversion chart to help guide you with approximate dose conversions when switching between thyroid hormone formulations. You can download this conversion chart from www.thyroidpharmacist.com/action.

4. Right Dose: Are You Taking the Right Amount?

Thyroid hormones are Goldilocks hormones, meaning the dose has to be "just right" for us to feel optimal. Patients are often underdosed on their thyroid medications and, in some cases, overdosed. Both scenarios result in unwanted symptoms.

"Start low and go slow" is a typical pharmacist mantra, and I like to recommend the same approach for thyroid medications. Usually the patient is started on a low-dose thyroid medication and the dose is gradually increased to normalize TSH, free T4, and free T3. This is to avoid shocking the body with a dramatic change and to determine the appropriate amount needed.

After a person is started on the initial dose, the thyroid function should be retested in four to six weeks, and the dose should be adjusted accordingly. This routine test-and-adjust cycle should be continued until the person's labs and symptoms are no longer indicating thyroid dysfunction.

While most doctors know to start their patients at a low dose, often the dose is not optimized. Many patients are underdosed and are only given enough thyroid hormone to move them from the overtly hypothyroid state to a slightly hypothyroid state. This is yet another reason why many continue to have symptoms despite taking medications!

While numbers are not the be-all and end-all, most of my readers and clients will report that they feel best with a TSH between 0.5 and 2 μIU/mL and when their free T3 and free T4 are in the top half of the reference range. Meanwhile, a TSH as high as 10 μIU/mL may be considered normal by some clinicians. And this is once again why I always recommend you get a copy of your lab results—don't just take your doctor's word for it—and do your own digging.

As you'll remember from chapter 2, when the "normal" ranges of TSH were originally set, they inadvertently included elderly patients and others with compromised thyroid function in the calculations, leading to an overly lax reference range. Consequently, many people with underactive thyroid hormones have been told that their thyroid tests were

SUMMARY OF THYROID MEDICATIONS

Brand Name (Generic Name)	Description
Armour Thyroid, Nature-Throid, WP Thyroid, NP Thyroid (thyroid USP)	Desiccated pork thyroid gland T4/T3 combination. Mimics the biological ratio of 80% T4 to 20% T3 with a T4:T3 ratio of 4:1. May also contain TPO and thyroglobulin, which can perpetuate the autoimmune attack in some. WP Thyroid is hypoallergenic.
Proloid (thyroglobulin)	Partially purified pork thyroglobulin. T4:T3 ratio of 2.5:1.
Synthroid, Levothyroid, Levoxyl, Thyro-Tabs, Uni-throid (levothyroxine)	Synthetic T4. Variable absorption among products. Should not switch back and forth between brand and generics.
Cytomel (liothyronine)	Synthetic T3.
Liotrix (thyrolar)	Synthetic T4:T3 in 4:1 ratio. Product on long-term back order at time of writing.
Compounded thyroid medications	Tailored dosage forms with a unique ratio of T4:T3 and free of allergenic fillers prepared by specialized compounding pharmacists. May be formulated as immediate-release or slow-release medications. Slow-release products may be more difficult to absorb.
Tirosint (levothyroxine)	New liquid gelcap formulation of T4; contains only glycerin, gelatin, and water. May be better absorbed and hypoallergenic. Less likely to interfere with coffee or proton pump inhibitors.

Second-Opinion Resources

If you continue to struggle with symptoms related to under-treatment of thyroid disease, it may be time for you to seek a second opinion from a doctor who is familiar with prescribing a variety of thyroid hormones and not just levothyroxine. I recommend that you use the practitioner database on my website as a starting point to finding a new doctor, and you can also work with your local compounding pharmacist (see the compounding pharmacy database on my website) to see if they have a recommendation for the most knowledgeable thyroid doctor in your area. You may be surprised that the doctors with the most positive feedback from the thyroid community may not be actual endocrinologists!

It's advisable that you call the doctor's office before you make your appointment to be sure they have experience with using a variety of thyroid medications. You can ask the staff if the doctor prescribes Armour Thyroid, Nature-Throid, WP Thyroid, compounded thyroid medications, Tirosint, or Cytomel.

Please go to www.thyroidpharmacist.com/action to gain access to the practitioner and compounding pharmacy databases.

normal even when they were not. It's important to remember that reference ranges may not be applicable to everyone and that you should take your symptoms into consideration as well as your lab results.

Of course, getting your lab results and understanding them are two different things. I always encourage my clients to become savvy at reading the lab results. While there are numerous thyroid lab tests that can be done, for the purposes of optimizing thyroid medications, the three most important lab tests are TSH, free T3, and free T4. Reverse T3 may also be used to determine if a person may

Root Cause Reflection:
Take Charge of Your Own Health!

Personally, I still have a copy of one of my TSH tests that showed a value of 4.5 µIU/mL with a note from the physician that said, "Your thyroid function is normal. No need to do anything." Meanwhile, I was sleeping twelve-plus hours per night and wearing sweaters in the middle of July in Southern California! I made the mistake of trusting another person with my health, and I lost a year of quality life because of it. Instead of pursuing my passions, I came home from work each day and collapsed. I don't want you to make the same mistake I did.

I encourage you to take charge of your own health. Learn as much as you can about your condition. Always request a copy of your labs. Don't be afraid to tell your doctor that you are not feeling well on current therapy, and insist on getting better care. There are plenty of doctors out there who will provide the care you need, so don't be afraid to seek out a second opinion.

How will you take charge of your own health today?

benefit from more T3. Use these tips as a general guide to understanding lab results:

- A TSH below 0.3 µIU/mL, with or without a free T3 or free T4 above the reference range, may suggest that you are overdosed on your medications.
- A TSH above 2 µIU/mL, with or without a free T3 or a free T4 below the reference range, may suggest that you are underdosed on your medications.

- In contrast, a TSH below 0.3 μIU/mL with a free T3 or a free T4 below the reference range may suggest a communication breakdown between the thyroid and the pituitary.
- When free T3 is below or within the low end of the reference range while free T4 is above the reference range or in the optimal upper part of the reference range, this suggests that a person may benefit from a T4/T3 combination medication due to impaired conversion.
- An elevated reverse T3 may suggest that a person may benefit from a higher dose of T3 while working on stress reduction and other triggers that may elevate reverse T3.

A note about labs: Thyroid medications containing T3 (Armour Thyroid, compounded T4/T3, Thyrolar, and Cytomel) can skew thyroid function test results, making people seem overdosed when they are indeed dosed correctly. When testing thyroid functions, tests should be done before the daily dose of medication is taken. As these medications are generally taken in the morning, individuals should postpone their medication until after the blood test has been performed.

Keep in mind that the levels that make each person feel their best are going to vary. Your optimal thyroid numbers are going to be different from your mother's optimal thyroid numbers, which are going to be different from your neighbor's optimal thyroid numbers. This is why it's so important for you to track your thyroid symptoms while taking thyroid medications, to determine your personal best.

Some doctors may be set in their ways, and just as they may not be willing to adjust your medication, they may not be willing to adjust your dose. They also may be wary of treating a person with a TSH below 10 μIU/mL. In that case, again, it's up to you to seek a second opinion.

Root Cause Research Corner: Survey Results from 2,232 People with Hashimoto's

Question: What is the optimal TSH range for you to feel your best?

ROOT CAUSE TSH SURVEY

TSH Range	Percentage Reported Feeling Better	Percentage Reported Feeling Worse	Percentage Did Not Notice Change
Under 1 µIU/ mL	70	12	18
Between 1 and 2 µIU/ mL	57	20	23
Above 2 µIU/ mL	10	67	23

A Caution About Overdosing

More is not always better! Doses that are too high can result in hyperthyroidism, which is dangerous and can lead to osteoporosis, anxiety, and cardiac problems. And we've already covered the concerns of undertreatment.

Please take the assessment below to ensure you are not experiencing any symptoms of over- or undertreatment. If you are experiencing symptoms of either, please talk to your doctor to have your thyroid levels tested.

I hope that by addressing the four Rs of optimal thyroid medication use, you will see an improvement in your hair, energy, and metabolism as well as any other residual symptoms you may be experiencing.

UNDERTREATMENT OR OVERTREATMENT ASSESSMENT

Mark which symptoms apply to you.

Symptoms of Undertreatment	Symptoms of Overtreatment
☐ Apathy	☐ Agitation
☐ Brain fog	☐ Excess sweating
☐ Cold intolerance	☐ Heat intolerance
☐ Eyebrow thinning/loss	☐ Insomnia
☐ Fatigue	☐ Irritability
☐ Hair loss	☐ Mood swings
☐ Heavy periods	☐ Palpitations
☐ Joint pain	☐ Rapid heart rate
☐ Puffy face	☐ Restlessness
☐ Sadness	☐ Scant periods
☐ Tangled hair	☐ Weight loss
☐ Weight gain	

If you still need help with adjusting your medications, you may benefit from unconventional medication protocols. Entire books have been written about thyroid medications. In fact, I've written a short book called *Optimizing Thyroid Medications* that takes a deep dive into various types of thyroid medications, medication protocols, medication titration, thyroid medication sensitivities, fillers, case studies, and much more. You can download a free copy of the e-book and access other tools at www.thyroidpharmacist.com/action.

Thinking Long Term: Medications and Thyroid Regeneration

Beyond helping you balance hormones through prescription medications, this chapter will also share methods that can support thyroid tissue regeneration, including low-level laser therapy, glandulars, and complementary aromatherapy protocols.

Most conventional medicine physicians and endocrinologists will say that in Hashimoto's, hypothyroidism is irreversible and ends with complete thyroid cell damage, leading to a lifelong requirement of thyroid hormone medications. In this scenario, Hashimoto's becomes a chronic condition, and care is dependent on the traditional medical system with ongoing physician visits, lab monitoring, and daily medication. The only change seen down the road is the dose escalation that will need to occur as thyroid tissue destruction worsens.

However, this isn't true! It has been reported that thyroid function spontaneously returned in 20 percent of patients with Hashimoto's. These individuals will return to normal thyroid function even after thyroid hormone replacement is withdrawn. Studies show that once the autoimmune attack ceases, the damaged thyroid has the ability to regenerate. Thyroid ultrasounds will show normal thyroid tissue that has regenerated, and the person will no longer test positive for TPO antibodies.

Lifestyle interventions can also help with reducing TPO antibodies, reversing hypothyroidism and Hashimoto's, and preventing other diseases—and they make most people feel better. Some may be able to reduce and eliminate the need for thyroid medications when the autoimmune attack ceases and the thyroid gland is able to regenerate. This regeneration may often be missed in adult patients because they are assumed to have hypothyroidism for life and antibodies and ultrasounds are not usually repeated after the initial diagnosis.

Despite the 20 percent spontaneous recovery rate, most physicians tell their patients thyroid medication is for life. Perhaps it is easier and less expensive to have someone on pills for life instead of running tests and attempting to taper down a medication.

Some people will present with hyperthyroidism as their bodies begin to heal and they absorb more of their thyroid medications or they produce more of their own hormones as thyroid tissue regenerates. Seeing a person with palpitations and a suppressed TSH will encourage most physicians to lower the dose of thyroid medications.

In other cases, even when the thyroid gland regenerates and could produce enough thyroid hormone without the need for a supplement, the medication can get built into our physiology due to hormonal feedback, and internal hormone synthesis turns off because there is enough supplemental hormone circulating. The recovery of thyroid function in these individuals becomes more difficult to catch. Physicians can perform thyroid ultrasounds to look for normalization of thyroid tissue as well as check for thyroid antibodies. If thyroid appearance on ultrasound normalizes and antibodies are in the remission range, a trial of slowly tapering thyroid medications may be attempted.

In addition to doing an ultrasound and checking TPO antibodies, another test can be done by administering TRH (thyrotropin-releasing hormone), which will cause an increase in T3 and T4 if the thyroid has recovered. While this test is the best way to determine if the person can be weaned off thyroid medications safely, it is rarely used in practice. Dr. Raphael Kellman in New York is a brilliant functional medicine doctor and one of the few doctors who utilize this test.

For those already taking thyroid supplements, it is crucial never to stop the medication abruptly. Abrupt cessation can lead to severe hypothyroid symptoms and cause a rapid escalation of TSH, leading to more thyroid damage. Gradual tapering of the medication is necessary and should only be done under the supervision of a physician.

Regaining Thyroid Function

While it's true that a damaged thyroid has the ability to regenerate once the disease is in remission, the rate of thyroid gland regeneration will vary with every person. Furthermore, while getting Hashimoto's into remission is generally considered a prerequisite for regenerating thyroid tissue, not every person who is in remission will have spontaneous tissue regeneration.

Therefore, even with all of your ducks in a row, not everyone will be able to reduce and eliminate the need for thyroid medications. Understandably, those who have had a full thyroidectomy will not be able to regenerate thyroid tissue, and generally the longer the person has had the condition and the more damage they've sustained, the longer and more difficult the regeneration of the thyroid tissue will be.

When it comes to accelerating thyroid tissue regeneration, I've had clients report results from four very different interventions: the immune-modulating medication naltrexone, low-level laser therapy (LLLT), glandulars, and complementary aromatherapy protocols. Let's explore.

Low-Dose Naltrexone

A book on Hashimoto's would not be complete if I didn't discuss the use of low-dose naltrexone (LDN).

Naltrexone is an FDA-approved medication used for opioid withdrawal at a dose of 50 mg per day. However, low doses of this medication have been found to modulate the immune system and have shown promise in improving cases of autoimmune disease, including Crohn's, multiple sclerosis, and Hashimoto's as well as other immune system–related conditions such as cancer and HIV/AIDS.

Doses of 1.5 to 4.5 mg every night at bedtime are usually recommended and have been reported to enhance immune function through increasing our endogenous endorphin production, reducing inflammation, promoting DNA synthesis, and slowing down motility in the GI tract to facilitate healing.

According to Dr. Kent Holtorf, LDN can improve the transport of thyroid hormones into cells, improve T4 to T3 conversion, and reduce the conversion of T4 to reverse T3.

My clients and readers have reported a reduction or elimination of thyroid symptoms, a reduction in thyroid antibodies (I have seen numbers as high as 1,000 IU/ml drop down into the <35 IU/ml range within a few months), improvement in the free T3 thyroid hormone levels, and in some cases a reduced need for thyroid medications with the use of LDN.

LDN will not work for everyone and should be combined with other functional medicine protocols for optimal benefit. In my Hashimoto's survey, 38 percent of those who tried LDN reported feeling better, and the ones who saw benefit had some spectacular results. Nearly 50 percent were able to reduce thyroid antibodies, 61 percent saw an improvement in mood, 66 percent had more energy, and 40 percent saw a reduction in pain.

One reader wrote: "Low-dose naltrexone changed my life for the better. If I had not added that to my regimen, I would still be suffering from nerve pain and uncontrollable allergy symptoms, in addition to the problems I have from the Hashimoto's."

As LDN can produce a rapid decline in autoimmunity, cases of hyperthyroidism necessitating a lowering of thyroid medications have been reported in people who have Hashimoto's and take thyroid medications. A starting dose of 0.5 mg is recommended in Hashimoto's, with periodic dosage increases of 0.5 mg until a target dose of 3 to 4.5 mg is reached.

This medication is available only as a prescription and can be compounded into lower doses by special professional compounding pharmacies. Luckily, even without insurance coverage, this medication is available in generic form and is very affordable, usually costing between $15 and $40 per month.

Best of all, in contrast to other medications, LDN has minimal side effects. The most common reported side effect is vivid dreaming, which is usually transient.

I recommend LDN for people who are looking to minimize their dose of thyroid medications, have multiple autoimmune conditions, experience multiple symptoms, have a high amount of thyroid antibodies, or report elusive root causes.

Low-Level Laser Therapy

LLLT is a clinically researched option for Hashimoto's that can regenerate thyroid tissue and reduce thyroid autoimmunity, restoring thyroid function! While most body organs are not accessible to laser therapy, the thyroid gland is close enough to the skin surface that the laser can penetrate it. Additionally, this therapy is painless, noninvasive, low cost, and low risk, as it does not use ionizing radiation.

Over the course of several studies, researchers in Brazil tested LLLT on patients who had Hashimoto's and were treated with levothyroxine. Patients received ten applications of LLLT (830 nm, output power 50nW) in continuous mode over the thyroid gland, twice per week for five weeks. Thirty days after the LLLT intervention, ultrasounds began to show improvements on the thyroid. Thyroid antibody levels began to decrease within two months of the LLLT, and thyroid function began to improve and continued to improve until it reached a peak at ten months post-treatment.

All of the patients were able to reduce their levothyroxine dose, and almost half (47 percent) did not need levothyroxine past the nine-month follow-up! The average levothyroxine dose dropped from 96 +/-22 mcg/day to 38 +/-23 mcg/day.

Overall, 95 percent of the study group had less thyroid damage and fewer attacking white blood cells after the treatment. Additionally, those with an enlarged or reduced thyroid gland saw that their thyroid size started to normalize, resulting in complete normalization in 43 percent! Thus this therapy may also be helpful for reducing autoimmunity conditions in the thyroid, decreasing thyroid antibodies, minimizing goiter size, and even normalizing a shrunken thyroid gland!

The researchers noted that the effects of the therapy may not last forever—a person may need to go in for maintenance treatment on a periodic basis. However, when used along with the Root Cause Approach of removing triggers, this therapy can potentially result in a functional cure of Hashimoto's for some people.

Please note, this therapy has not been tested on people who take immunosuppressants like corticosteroids, people with thyroid nodules, people with hypothyroidism from postpartum thyroiditis, or people with Graves' disease. At present, this therapy is still considered experimental and is not FDA approved—however, individual doctors may be able to utilize this therapy with their patients as an "off-label" use.

I have been working with laser companies, clinicians, and research institutions to attempt to facilitate the introduction of this therapy into the United States and Europe. While we're making progress, the process has been slow and challenging. I'm pleased to announce that at the time of writing this book, Dr. Kirk Gair from West Covina, California, who is also a Hashimoto's patient, has used cold lasers in his clinic since 2004 and has developed protocols that combine LLLT with functional medicine modalities. He is also working to train other practitioners and spread awareness about LLLT with autoimmune thyroid disease. For updates and a listing of clinicians who specialize in LLLT, please be sure to go to www.thyroidpharmacist. com/action.

Nonprescription Thyroid Glandulars

Some thyroid glandulars (products isolated from the thyroid glands of animals) have been reported to help with regenerating thyroid tissue. This could be due to materials present in these extracts that contain messenger chemicals that encourage tissue regeneration.

While not all glandulars are created equally, I've seen positive results with Thytrophin PMG from Standard Process, while my colleague Dr. Kelly Brogan has had positive results from Thyroid Natural Glandular from Allergy Research Group.

Thyroid patients have reported a reduction in symptoms, a reduction in thyroid antibodies, and an improvement in thyroid hormone levels on lab tests. Additionally, some have reported utilizing these products for a six- to twelve-month period that allowed them to normalize their TSH and subsequently allowed them to discontinue the glandular while their thyroid hormone levels remained optimal.

These options may be especially interesting for patients who are unable to find doctors to prescribe NDT medications, those with only a slight elevation in TSH, or those who did not tolerate thyroid medications. If you are considering using glandulars, please consult with a practitioner before combining them with thyroid medications.

Aromatherapy and Essential Oils

If you've been trained or indoctrinated in conventional medicine like I have, you'll likely be skeptical about the use of essential oils. Although I have always been interested in pharmacognosy, or synthesizing medicines from plants—after all, our first medicines came from roots and herbs, not from laboratories—using flower essences to treat "real" health conditions seemed a little far-fetched.

I became more interested in aromatherapy after hearing from a couple of my clients who reported a reduction in thyroid antibodies and thyroid medications with the use of frankincense oil.

Aromatherapy, as a healing modality, derives much of its perceived benefit from the scent of the essential oils, which results in a response from the brain that changes the body's setting. Think of a time when you smelled some fragrant flowers—if you're like most people, the thought alone will boost your mood and help you feel more relaxed. As we know, stress is a big trigger in autoimmune disease, so it's easy to see how even that subtle change in mood can have a positive effect on the thyroid and adrenals.

Upon deeper investigation, one will learn that the use of essential oils does have some additional merit. Essential oils contain active substances with pharmacological activity that are absorbed when the oils are applied to the skin, inhaled, or ingested. While I would never tell someone to stop taking their medications and replace them with essential oils, I think essential oils are a wonderful *complementary* therapy that can be utilized in conjunction with the other interventions you are incorporating (plus, they smell great and can be used as a replacement for toxic perfumes).

Essential oils can be diffused in the air with an oil diffuser, taken internally, or applied topically. One of my colleagues Carrie

Vitt swears by using a blend of essential oils like frankincense, clove, myrrh, marjoram, basil, and lemongrass applied topically to the thyroid gland to support thyroid function naturally. Myrtle and lavender (*Lavandula angustifolia* not *Lavandula* × *intermedia*) may also help. Myrtle is a potent adaptogen. Lavender helps with restoring hair and calming anxiety.

Caution should be exercised when using essential oils. Please keep the following in mind if you're thinking about incorporating essential oils to your routine:

- Many oils need to be properly diluted with carrier oils like coconut oil or jojoba oil before applied to the skin to prevent irritation.
- I don't advise ingesting essential oils internally unless you're working with a qualified aromatherapist, as some oils may be toxic when taken internally.

Weaning Thyroid Medications

Thyroid medications should never be stopped abruptly due to the complicated feedback mechanisms of our hormones. You want to give your body an opportunity to slowly get used to producing thyroid hormones—thus thyroid medications should be reduced very gradually under the supervision of a physician and supported by lab tests. An initial dose reduction of 25 mcg equivalents of levothyroxine can be initiated to determine if thyroid regeneration has occurred, and lab tests should be done four to six weeks later to ensure that the person's thyroid function remains normal. If the thyroid function remains normal, another equivalent dose reduction may be attempted, followed by testing in another four to six weeks.

Final Thoughts on Optimizing Thyroid Hormones

Once you optimize your thyroid hormones, you'll find that you will have more energy, an ability to tolerate cold, and a better mood within a few days. Your weight will also begin to optimize within a few weeks. Hair loss will resolve in four to eight weeks and will be followed by hair regrowth approximately eight to twelve weeks after medication optimization. Furthermore, many have reported the resolution of strange, seemingly unrelated symptoms like anxiety, bladder spasms, carpal tunnel, and many others. Optimizing thyroid hormones is an important part of regaining your health, and I hope that this chapter has given you some strategies to implement while working with your practitioner.

9

Protocols for Mastering
Nutrition and Nutrients

I f you've arrived at this Advanced Protocol, you likely have some unresolved symptoms that could be related to outstanding nutrient deficiencies or food reactions. In this chapter, I'll share with you some ways to address these issues that could be interfering with your recovery from Hashimoto's.

Before we get into these advanced strategies, I want to address some dangerous diet dogmas that can also interfere with healing. Understanding these dogmas will help you avoid unnecessary delays in your recovery from Hashimoto's.

Dangerous Diet Dogmas

Dogma #1: Diet can heal everything. If I just take out more foods, I will be healed. While some people have had great success through changing their diets, even going into complete remission from Hashimoto's, diet changes alone may not be enough in many cases. Eating a nutrient-dense diet that is free of reactive foods can do wonders, and it's one of the first things I recommend, but if you've been on a clean diet for three months and you're not seeing results or are getting stuck, you likely have an unwanted guest that is living inside of you and causing inflammation within your body.

This guest may be a toxin or a pathogen like a parasite or a bacterial overgrowth. While people are open to the presence of toxins, many find the suggestion of parasites alarming. However, these are more common than you think when it comes to gut infections and factors preventing a person from healing. In 2015, 80 percent of my clients who did not go into remission with nutrition alone tested positive for one or more gut infections. Gut infections lead to intestinal permeability, which, as you know, is one of the main triggers of Hashimoto's. Most infections require targeted treatments such as herbs, antibiotics, antifungals, or antiprotozoal agents in order to be eradicated. No amount of food restriction will heal an infection, and when you have an infection, you will be sensitive to whatever you're eating (see chapter 11).

Dogma #2: Reducing calories and increasing my exercise are the keys to weight loss with thyroid disease. This dogma may have been reinforced by various doctors who perhaps said you have fork-to-mouth syndrome. Unfortunately, this extreme calorie restriction (with or without exercise) is not just unkind, but it can also put your body into an adaptive physiology mode of conserving calories as though you were in a famine, worsening your hypothyroidism and adrenal dysfunction, and preventing effortless weight loss that occurs once we're nutrient sufficient.

Dogma #3: All nutrients should be obtained from food. Some idealists may say that we should get all of our nutrients from foods, but that's not always possible, especially for people with Hashimoto's who have multiple food sensitivities, nutrient-depleting infections, and digestive difficulties. Furthermore, our current food supply is not as nutrient rich as it was in decades past due to soil depletion and conventional farming practices. Additionally, some symptoms and conditions can benefit from megadosing nutrients in quantities that you would not find in foods. This is why I frequently recommend supplements to address outstanding symptoms.

In the following pages, I'll introduce some ways to address these issues that could be interfering with your recovery from Hashimoto's. I'm going to share more tools and tips for dialing in your nutrition based on your unique symptoms, food sensitivities, infections, or toxins that may be present within your body.

Advanced Dietary Modifications to Help You Heal from Hashimoto's

I could write an entire series of books on dietary modifications alone, and most of the information is readily available on the internet, so in the interest of space, I'm going to provide guidance on the top five modifications I recommend. For additional guidance on dietary modifications, please go to www.thyroidpharmacist.com/action.

Modification #1: Additional Food Sensitivity Testing

When we have intestinal permeability, there's a chance that we can become sensitized to just about every food out there! We've already eliminated the top reactive foods in the Fundamental Protocols, but some people may still have outstanding foods that are causing a reaction. I generally recommend elimination diets like the Root Cause Intro, Root Cause Paleo, and Root Cause Autoimmune Diets I introduced in the Fundamental Protocols to figure out your unique sensitivities rather than doing food sensitivity testing. This is because no food sensitivity tests are as accurate as your own body in detecting the reactions you may have to foods.

Food sensitivity tests can have false positives and false negatives alike. On one hand, I've seen people with needlessly restricted diets because their food sensitivity analyses tested for multiple reactive pathways and deemed most foods as reactive. On the other hand, many other people have delayed their healing by continuing to eat gluten because a food sensitivity test didn't report a reaction even though gluten is reactive in close to 90 percent of people with Hashimoto's.

Of course I've found that there are certain tests that tend to be more accurate than others for food sensitivity testing. I'll share the tests I have found to be the most beneficial, but first, I'd like to highlight a couple of situations in which food sensitivity tests are recommended:

- **When someone is already eating a diet like the Root Cause Paleo Diet or Root Cause Autoimmune Diet, yet they still continue to have symptoms:** This is especially the case if the symptoms are food sensitivity reactions such as breakouts, bloating, fatigue, or headaches that occur after meals. In some cases, the cause might be unusual-suspect foods like citrus fruit, peaches, or pineapples that are not always easy to identify through a traditional elimination diet. These types of reactions are usually temporary and resolve once the gut is healed; however, eliminating them in the short term for three to six months can produce a profound improvement on symptoms.
- **When a person needs to see their results on paper to make a change:** I get it; I was one of those people, and forking out money on tests motivated me to make a commitment to adhere to the test results.

Types of Tests to Get

I remember telling a colleague at work how food sensitivity testing helped me uncover a sensitivity to dairy and that getting off that food made my acid reflux go away. Excited, my colleague went to see his allergist and had him order an allergy test. Unfortunately, the test didn't reveal any reactive foods. As discussed earlier, this is because the tests done by allergists analyze for food *allergies*, which are governed by the IgE branch of the immune system. Food *sensitivities*, though similar sounding, are a different type of immune reaction governed by the IgG or sometimes the IgA and IgM branch of the immune system. Food allergies are widely accepted as true medical conditions by conventional practitioners, while food sensitivities are considered experimental and not recognized by conventional medicine or insurance companies.

In Hashimoto's, I'm specifically interested in IgG food sensitivity testing. IgG food reactions are known as type IV hypersensitivity reactions. Hashimoto's, too, seems to be governed (at least partially) by the IgG branch of the immune system and is considered a type IV hypersensitivity reaction. Though there is no research supporting this yet, anecdotally, I have seen that eating IgG reactive foods does seem to fuel Hashimoto's.

If you're looking for a specific brand of IgG test, at the time of writing this book, I've found that the Alletess food sensitivity test has been the most accurate for my clients and myself. If a food comes up positive on that test, I know that it is most likely a reactive food for that person. In some cases, especially if the person has been off the foods for some time, this test may produce false negatives. If a false negative comes for one of the big reactive foods, I still recommend that the person eliminate the food for a minimum of three weeks, then attempt a reintroduction to determine if a reaction occurs. If you've been off a food and feel better, I recommend waiting for three to six months before attempting a reintroduction.

If you are working with an integrative and functional medicine physician, you can ask them to order the Alletess test. If not, I'm excited to tell you that I finally have an option that people can self-order without a prescription. This is something I've coordinated with a direct-to-patient lab, and the test kit can be done in your own home, just about anywhere in the world. I recommend repeating this test on an annual basis. Our food sensitivities and reactions to foods can change with time, so I have found that annual testing helps me stay on top or ahead of my potential triggers.

The lab will also send me updates on the most reactive foods for people with Hashimoto's who have gotten the tests so that I'll be able to share this information with you in future newsletters. For more information, please go to www.thyroidpharmacist.com/action.

Modification #2: Carbohydrate Intake

If you are an athlete or find yourself more tired on the traditional Paleo or Autoimmune Paleo diets, or if you have excess cortisol, elevated reverse T3, and hormonal abnormalities, you may benefit from getting more carbohydrates. Rather than filling up on processed grains, I recommend adding more real food carbohydrates, such as pumpkin, squash (butternut squash is an excellent choice), sweet potatoes, plantains, bananas, apples, cassava flour, legumes, and grain-like seeds such as buckwheat, quinoa, or white rice (as long as you're not sensitive).

Please note, some people report feeling tired after starting a protein- and fat-heavy diet like the Paleo diet, but this is not always due to a reduced intake of carbohydrates. In fact, some people with autoimmune disease and Hashimoto's feel amazing on a strict low-carb, ketogenic diet. If you're feeling tired on a diet that is mostly composed of fats and proteins, this could be due to low stomach acid, which leads to improper protein digestion.

In the Gut Balance Protocol, I discussed the fact that most people with Hashimoto's have low stomach acid, which impairs our ability to digest protein foods. People who are low in stomach acid may find themselves naturally gravitating toward carbohydrates for energy, as carbohydrates do not need as much digestive juice as proteins for proper digestion.

If you have continued to eat a high-carbohydrate diet because you suspect you need more carbs for energy, I encourage you to revisit the Gut Balance Protocol, specifically the section on the digestive enzyme betaine with pepsin. This should absolutely be included in your supplement regimen before you determine if low carb is a good choice for you. Many people have found that taking this supplement helped with fatigue. Other options for increasing stomach acid and improving digestion include hot lemon water or a teaspoon of apple cider vinegar in a glass of water with protein-containing meals.

Modification #3: Real Food Smoothies

When a person begins to eat all real foods, this unmasks something we don't see often with our modern diet due to the bulking effects of grains and hormones in dairy: malabsorption and poor nutrient assimilation. These conditions will lead to a person becoming underweight. Some of the root causes of this may be impaired cortisol production (see chapter 10), gut infections like SIBO or parasites (see chapter 11), overmedication (see chapter 8), nutrient depletions, or an inadequate calorie intake due to maladjusted satiety signaling that develops after a lifetime of eating nutrient-poor foods.

To determine if you are indeed eating enough calories, get a calorie-counting app, such as MyFitnessPal, on your phone to help you keep track of your daily calories. Eating real food can be more filling than eating simple carbohydrates so you may feel full but not be getting enough calories. The app will help you to figure out your target weight (whether you want to lose or gain weight) and the number of calories per day you need to get there.

In order to increase your weight, I recommend adding the Modified Root Cause Build Smoothie *after dinner* as you work out your other root causes. Smoothies are better absorbed and can be filled with quality calories. When consuming the smoothies after dinner, rather than at breakfast, you won't set off our body's full signals for the day. When you have a smoothie in the morning, however, it will keep you full all day, so you may opt for having real food in the morning and smoothies at bedtime if you're trying to gain weight.

Modified Root Cause Build Smoothie

1 avocado

1 cup coconut milk

1 banana

2 egg yolks (if tolerated)

1 scoop hydrolyzed beef protein

Add ingredients to a blender and blend thoroughly. You can add water to thin out the consistency, which will make it easier to eat and feel less filling. This is a great way to add 700+ calories to your daily intake. You can also add cooked sweet potatoes if you need more carbs or calories to meet your goal.

Modification #4: Iodine Intake

I mentioned that iodine excess has been recognized as a trigger to Hashimoto's. This is true particularly in people who are genetically predisposed to Hashimoto's and who may perhaps have certain vulnerabilities like a selenium deficiency.

If you have been exposed to high doses of iodine, it may be helpful to take a selenium supplement, up to 400 mcg per day, to negate the negative effects of the iodine excess.

In some cases, a low-iodine diet has been helpful in reducing the autoimmune attack on the thyroid gland and in normalizing thyroid function in people with iodine-induced Hashimoto's. In this case, a person would temporarily restrict iodine to less than 100 mcg per day for a period of one to three months (the thyroid gland needs approximately 52 mcg per day of iodine, which is usually present in thyroid hormones, which contain a small amount of iodine). This would mean limiting your intake of iodine from supplements as well as high-iodine-containing foods like seaweed, kelp, spirulina, chlorella, and even seafood. For more information about the low-iodine approach, please see my first book, *Hashimoto's Thyroiditis: Lifestyle Interventions for Finding and Treating the Root Cause.*

Modification #5: Root Cause Rotation Diet

The Root Cause Rotation Diet is helpful for people who have multiple food sensitivities and symptoms but have not found relief from the Root Cause Intro, Paleo, or Autoimmune Diets. This diet is also for those who keep losing foods, becoming sensitive to more and more foods as time goes on, or have multiple autoimmune conditions.

Root Cause Research Corner:
Iodine—a Very Controversial Root Cause

If you've looked up thyroid disorders on the internet, chances are that you found some contradictory information about the role of iodine in thyroid health. Some health experts claim that iodine deficiency is the cause of thyroid disorders and that iodine supplements will resolve them. Others say that iodine excess can cause thyroid disorders and that taking iodine will make them worse. Where's the truth? Somewhere in the middle! Iodine is an important component of thyroid hormones, and iodine deficiency can result in hypothyroidism. However, Hashimoto's thyroiditis is not typically associated with iodine deficiency. In fact, iodine excess has been recognized as a trigger in Hashimoto's.

Iodine has a narrow therapeutic index, where doses that are too low are problematic, leading to iodine-deficiency hypothyroidism, but doses that are too high can cause or exacerbate Hashimoto's!

This has to do with the way that iodine from foods and supplements is processed by the thyroid gland so that the body can properly use it. During this process, hydrogen peroxide—a free radical—is released. In cases when the body has adequate levels of selenium, and the selenium is used properly, it neutralizes the hydrogen peroxide. However, in cases of iodine excess, hydrogen peroxide can cause oxidative damage to the thyroid gland.

Studies have shown that excess iodine causes thyroid injury by generating reactive oxygen species—chemicals that lead to premature damage and programmed cell death in thyroid tissues. These iodine-overloaded cells then release the damage-associated, or danger-associated, molecular patterns (DAMPs) that turn on the autoimmune process in a person with genetic predisposition and intestinal permeability. When we think about this from an evolutionary, adaptive, or even innate body wisdom stance, this makes sense that the body would want to stop the production of excess thyroid hormones that would result from too much iodine.

Taking a high dose of iodine can exacerbate Hashimoto's and accelerate thyroid cell destruction. The American Thyroid Association cautions against using doses of more than 500 mcg per day and notes that doses above 1,100 mcg may cause thyroid dysfunction. These warnings are for the general population, but studies have found that people with Hashimoto's may be sensitive to even smaller doses.

While some thyroid advocates propose that taking high doses of iodine is helpful for everyone with a thyroid disorder, I have not seen this to be the case in Hashimoto's. I have seen an emergence of new thyroid symptoms and people's TSH and rates of thyroid antibodies dramatically increase as their thyroid hormone levels plummeted following the use of high doses of iodine. Dr. Datis Kharrazian, one of the world's foremost authorities on nondrug therapies for Hashimoto's, reports that iodine may increase the rates of not just thyroid antibodies but also brain antibodies, which may be seen in some people with Hashimoto's, leading to increased brain damage.

Out of my Root Cause readers who were surveyed, 356 tried high-dose iodine. Out of that group, 25 percent said high-dose iodine made them feel better, 28.5 percent said it made them feel worse, and 46.5 percent saw no difference in how they felt, although this doesn't mean that their thyroid markers weren't affected. The takeaway from this survey is that more people felt worse on high-dose iodine than felt better. On the other hand, iodine restriction made 32 percent feel better and 7 percent feel worse.

In contrast, taking a selenium supplement helped 63 percent feel better, 34 percent saw no difference, while 3 percent felt worse. Going gluten-free helped 88 percent of people feel better, 11 percent saw no difference, and 1 percent felt worse.

As you can see, there are many safer and much more effective interventions than iodine supplementation in Hashimoto's, which is why I have chosen to focus on the interventions that are helpful to most people and least likely to result in harm. I treat iodine like a narrow therapeutic drug and recommend caution with using it in Hashimoto's.

While there is a bit of controversy about whether people with Hashimoto's should take iodine or avoid it altogether, a 1999 study that followed 377 people with Hashimoto's for over eight hundred days found that when combined with thyroid hormone therapy, a daily iodine dose of up to 200 mcg per day was well tolerated and even reduced thyroid antibody levels.

For most people with Hashimoto's, I do not recommend doses above the recommended daily allowance (RDA) of iodine of 150 mcg for nonpregnant adults and 220 mcg and 290 mcg for pregnant and breastfeeding women, respectively. Doses as low as 300 mcg per day have the potential to exacerbate Hashimoto's.

It's important to remember that iodine is a Goldilocks nutrient, where just the right amounts are needed for optimal health.

In chapter 9, you'll find more details on how to address iodine toxicity and what to do if you were exposed to excessive doses. You can also check out my first book, *Hashimoto's Thyroiditis: Lifestyle Interventions for Finding and Treating the Root Cause,* for a comprehensive review of iodine in Hashimoto's and a protocol on iodine restriction.

The main focus of the Root Cause Rotation Diet is giving yourself twenty-four hours to enjoy foods within specific food families and then not having the foods again until four days later (see chart on facing page). Eating a food only once every four days can help reduce food reactions, prevent food sensitivities, and accelerate healing.

The food days can be assigned to each calendar day (you would be eating the designated day 1 foods for breakfast, lunch, and dinner on Monday, for example) or to each twenty-four-hour period for convenience and variety. (In this scenario, you would eat the designated day 1 foods for dinner on Monday, and also for breakfast and lunch on Tuesday. Day 2 foods would be eaten for Tuesday's dinner.)

The Root Cause Rotation Diet should be followed for thirty to ninety days while working to resolve advanced triggers. Please remember that dieting alone will not heal the gut!

FOOD FAMILIES TO FULLY EXCLUDE ON THE ROOT CAUSE ROTATION DIET

Caffeine

Dairy

Eggs

Grains

Legumes

Nightshades

Nuts

Seaweed

Seeds

Sugar

The most reactive foods are excluded from the Root Cause Rotation Diet. However, additional foods may need to be excluded per the results of your Alletess food sensitivity test or elimination diet. Keep in mind that some foods cross-react with other families—for example, a person who is almond sensitive may also cross-react with apricots, cherries, nectarines, peaches, plums, raisins, and prunes. A person who is sensitive to dates may also react to coconut and hearts of palms and vice versa.

For more Root Cause Rotation Diet resources, visit www.thyroid pharmacist.com/action. There you'll find recipes, meal plans, and shopping ideas.

ROOT CAUSE ROTATION DIET

Foods are grouped by "families," and the same families are eaten only every fourth day to minimize inflammation due to reactions.

Food Category	Day 1	Day 2	Day 3	Day 4
Vegetables	Sweet potato, yam, sorrel, mushroom, okra, asparagus, green beans	Arugula, broccoli, Brussels sprouts, cabbage, cauliflower, collard greens, daikon, kale, radish, watercress, hearts of palm	Pumpkin, squash, bitter melon, cucumber, zucchini, carrots, celery, fennel, parsley, parsnip, olives	Plantain, avocado, artichokes, dandelion, endive, lettuce, beets, chard, lamb's-quarters, spinach
Meat, fish, fowl	Beef, bison, buffalo, goat, lamb, duck, goose, deer, elk, rabbit, squab	Anchovy, catfish, cod, flounder, grouper, halibut, salmon, sardine, snapper, swordfish, tuna	Chicken, turkey, crab, lobster, shrimp	Clams, scallops, perch, trout, sole, whitefish, pork

Food Category	Day 1	Day 2	Day 3	Day 4
Fruit	Rhubarb, blueberry, cranberry, kiwi, persimmon, apricot, cherry, nectarine, peach, plum	Grapefruit, lemon, lime, mandarin, orange, tangerine, pineapple, grapes	Mango, cantaloupe, honeydew melon, elderberry, papaya, pomegranate	Banana, fig, mulberry, apple, pear, blackberry, raspberry, strawberry
Nuts/seeds		Coconut		
Thickeners	Yam puree, sweet potato puree		Squash puree, arrowroot	Applesauce
Drinks	Hibiscus tea	Lemon water, coconut water	Ginger tea, mint	Chamomile, chicory, dandelion root coffee
Spices	Garlic, leek, onion, shallot, vanilla, black pepper	Tamarind, carob, horseradish, mustard, wasabi, allspice, cloves	Cardamom, ginger, turmeric, anise, caraway, chervil, cilantro, coriander, cumin, dill, basil, marjoram, mint, oregano, rosemary, thyme	Capers, saffron, bay leaf, cinnamon, tarragon
Sweetener	Honey, prunes	Dates	Maple syrup	Black currant, stevia

Food Category	Day 1	Day 2	Day 3	Day 4
Fats and oils	Duck fat, goose fat	Coconut oil	Chicken fat, olive oil	Avocado oil, safflower oil, lard
Sour	Cranberry juice	Lemon juice, sauerkraut	Pickles, pomegranate	Apple cider vinegar, beet kvass

Root Cause Rotation Diet Meal Ideas

Meal Type	Day 1	Day 2	Day 3	Day 4
Breakfast	Beef hash with sweet potatoes, onions, leeks, and garlic, or leftovers from previous day	Stir-fried fish with kale, or leftovers from previous day	Turkey sausage with parsnip puree	Pork cutlets with avocado and artichokes or leftovers from previous day
Lunch	Portabella mushroom bison burgers with sweet potato fries	Halibut with Brussels sprouts puree	Turkey meatballs with spaghetti squash	Capers, saffron, and scallops over a bed of spinach
Dinner	Baked duck with plum sauce and steamed asparagus	Salmon with broccoli and mashed cauliflower	Chicken stew with squash and carrots	Pulled pork, plantains, and avocado
Snacks	Beef jerky and blueberries	Sardines, dried coconut flakes	Olives and pickles, papaya	Avocado with beets, plum sauce

Additional Modifications for Specific Symptoms

The Root Cause dietary modifications, including those introduced in the Fundamental Protocols (Root Cause Intro, Paleo, and Autoimmune Diets) and the one you just learned about in this chapter (Root Cause Rotation Diet), are based on my personal experience with numerous diets and clinical experience with my clients. These diets are meant to be a starting point for you and may need to be tailored to your individual needs and response.

Your personal combination of your ethnic background, current health status, environment, stress levels, infections, toxin exposure, and symptoms can further guide your dietary modifications. Here are some specific dietary modifications you can consider based on your symptoms or underlying triggers:

- **Fructose malabsorption or blood sugar abnormalities:** Reduce fructose intake to less than 50 g per day.
- **SIBO:** You may benefit from a low-FODMAP diet for two to six months, an elemental diet where meals are replaced by predigested macro- and micronutrients (Physicians' Elemental Diet by Integrative Therapeutics brand is the meal replacement I recommend) for two to three weeks, or a diet without fermented foods.
- **Symptoms of copper toxicity** (such as acne and hormonal breakouts, fatigue, emotional lability, and a reddish tint to your hair): Consider a low-copper diet. See page 346 for more information.
- **Symptoms of citrus sensitivity** (such as fatigue, allergies, headaches, sinus issues, rashes, and upset stomach): Remove citrus fruit.
- **For impaired detoxification:** Try a two-week vegan or vegetarian diet.
- **If you have lost too much weight:** Add the Modified Root Cause Build Smoothie to your diet (see page 265).
- *Candida:* Try a yeast-limiting diet like the Body Ecology Diet.

- **Neurological issues** (such as depression, anxiety, brain fog, epilepsy, pain, or migraines): A ketogenic diet—a low-carb diet where the body breaks down fats for fuel instead of relying on carbohydrates—could be beneficial.
- **Iodine toxicity** (after past exposure to high doses of iodine): A low-iodine diet for one to three months will help you recover.
- **Sulfur toxicity** (with symptoms such as dry skin, breakouts, and rashes): A low-sulfur diet can help eliminate symptoms. See page 345 for more information on the low-sulfur diet.
- **Mercury toxicity:** Follow a low-seafood diet.
- **Severe dairy reactions** (and are still experiencing symptoms): Consider a trial beef avoidance, which may also help reduce pain.
- **Inflammatory issues** (such as pain, vulvodynia, fibromyalgia, urinary burning, kidney stones, and irritable bladder not resolved by other diets or interventions): Follow a low-oxalate diet.
- **Malabsorption:** Consider reducing raw foods and try pureeing foods.
- **Impaired detoxification:** Increase your intake of raw foods.
- **Gallbladder issues:** Remove eggs, pork, onions, chicken, coffee, oranges, beans, nuts, apples, and tomatoes.
- **Mold toxicity:** Exclude high-mold foods and beverages such as peanuts, raisins, dried fruit, nuts, coffee, beer, and wine, and consider a low-mold diet like the Bulletproof Diet.

If you follow one of the above recommendations that requires the removal or elimination of a certain food or foods, you'll want to test it to see if that's what's causing your symptoms. To do this, remove all sources of the food for three weeks, observing symptoms throughout, and then reintroduce the food by eating it during three consecutive days. Observe your symptoms over these three days to determine if the food was indeed reactive.

Most of the symptom-based dietary modifications should be followed from two weeks to three months. In the initial stages of healing, we take away foods; as you begin to heal, you will be able to add in more and more foods. While people with Hashimoto's may start off with multiple food sensitivities, most will end up with three or fewer food sensitivities when in remission. Your needs may also change as time goes on, as you get rid of infections, or when you balance your intestinal flora.

For most people, a maintenance diet (after they've completed the Fundamental Protocols) will be a diet like the full Paleo diet or a diet that is gluten-free, dairy-free, and soy-free. Some individuals have been able to reintroduce all foods after they've reached remission; however, most will benefit from long-term abstaining of at minimal gluten. At present time, I suggest all those with autoimmune thyroid disease to consider lifelong removal of gluten, dairy, and soy.

Mastering Nutrients

In this section, I'll show you how to optimize your nutrient levels through the use of supplements. Some nutrients can be easily added to your regimen without worrying about test buildup in the body, while others will require assessments, testing, and special precautions.

The following symptoms may suggest additional needs for the associated vitamins or minerals, or the use of megadoses of vitamins or minerals:

- **Menstrual cramps, migraines, restless leg syndrome, constipation, anxiety:** You may benefit from magnesium citrate.
- **Muscle wasting:** You can benefit from a potassium bicarbonate supplement, a magnesium supplement, a multivitamin supplement like Nutrient 950 (iodine-, iron-, and copper-free) from Pure Encapsulations, and an amino acid powder like Amino-NR from Pure Encapsulations.
- **Pain, inflammation, dry skin, oily hair, acne, eczema:** You may benefit from 1–4 g of fish oil per day.
- **Fatigue, brain fog, low blood pressure, adrenal issues,**

carbohydrate intolerance: You may benefit from 600 mg of thiamine per day or more.

- **Vertigo, seizures, *H. pylori* infection, history of vegan or vegetarian diet:** Try methylcobalamin sublingual tablets, liquid vitamin B_{12}, or B_{12} injections (testing of levels recommended before supplementing).

- **Epstein-Barr virus, swollen glands, frequent colds:** You may benefit from 500–3,000 mg of vitamin C per day, or IV vitamin C.

- **Postpartum, breastfeeding, pregnancy, low reverse T3, adverse reaction to selenium, fibrocystic breasts:** You may benefit from an iodine supplement of up to 200 mcg per day.

- **Fat malabsorption** (greasy, floating, or light-colored stools, gas or belching, dry skin, gallbladder pain, gallstones, gallbladder removal, nausea, hormonal imbalances, vitamin ADEK deficiency): You may benefit from the Rootcology Liver & Gallbladder Support, the Digestion GB supplement from Pure Encapsulations, or the LV-GB supplement from Designs for Health.

- **Pancreatic enzyme insufficiency** (weight loss, diarrhea, gas, oily stools, bloating, stomach pain a few hours after eating): You may benefit from the Rootcology Liver & Gallbladder Support, Pancreatic Enzyme Formula from Pure Encapsulations, or the LV-GB supplement from Designs for Health.

- **Skin rashes, dryness, breakouts associated with sulfur sensitivity:** You may benefit from zinc picolinate doses above 30 mg and 100–600 mcg of molybdenum per day.

- **Fat malabsorption, living in a northern climate, low intake of fatty fish, low exposure to sunlight, history of Hashimoto's:** These suggest the need for vitamin D (testing of levels recommended before supplementing).

- **Hair loss, anemia, pale skin, fatigue, ice cravings, carrot cravings:** These suggest the need for ferritin or iron (testing of levels recommended before supplementing).

Food Reintroduction Chart

As you begin to reintroduce foods back into your life, here are some symptoms that could suggest you are reacting to a food and may need to exclude it for three to twelve months.

MANIFESTATIONS OF FOOD REACTIONS IN BODY SYSTEMS

System	Symptom
Respiratory	Postnasal drip, congestion, cough, asthma symptoms
Gastrointestinal	Constipation, diarrhea, cramping, bloating, nausea, gas, acid reflux, burning, burping
Cardiovascular	Increased pulse, palpitations
Skin	Acne, eczema, itchiness
Musculoskeletal	Joint aches, pain, swelling, tingling, numbness
Mental	Headache, dizziness, brain fog, anxiety, depression, fatigue, insomnia

Fundamental Nutrient Testing

I've already discussed testing for B_{12}, ferritin, and vitamin D in the Fundamental Protocols. Here is some more information on addressing ferritin and B_{12}.

Ferritin

Ferritin is the name given to your body's iron reserve protein. Ferritin is required for transport of T3 to cell nuclei and for the utilization of the T3 hormone. Ferritin deficiency can result in fatigue, cold intolerance, breathlessness, tongue abnormalities, and hair loss. Ferritin hair loss presents as increased hair loss during shampooing and brushing as well as overall thinning of hair without a specific pattern or bald spots. This means you'll find that your hair feels thinner all over and is less dense.

Ferritin levels can also be measured and will be a better predictor of how much iron you have stored in your body and available for use. Ferritin should be checked in all women with Hashimoto's and in anyone experiencing hair loss.

Normal ferritin levels for women are between 12 and 150 ng/mL. According to some experts, ferritin levels of at least 40 ng/mL are required to stop hair loss, while levels of at least 70 ng/mL are needed for hair regrowth. The optimal ferritin level for thyroid function is between 90 and 110 ng/mL.

Iron from foods comes in two types: the heme and nonheme versions. The heme version is better absorbed and is found primarily in animal products. The highest levels of iron are found in organ meats … yes, delicious liver. Beef, turkey, and chicken are the next best choices. (Sorry to all of my vegetarian friends.) In contrast, nonheme iron is found in nuts, beans, and spinach and is not usually absorbed as well.

To restore your iron levels, you can eat cooked liver twice per week or beef a few times per week. Vitamin C increases the absorption of iron, so taking a vitamin C tablet or eating a vitamin C–rich food such as cooked broccoli along with an iron-rich food is the best way to increase iron and ferritin levels. Creating an acidic stomach environment by taking a betaine with pepsin supplement with meals can be helpful as well.

You can also take iron supplements. However, most of them are in the nonheme form and may not be absorbed well. Additionally, many people find that they get terrible stomachaches from the supplements, and they find them extremely constipating!

If choosing to take iron supplements, do so with much caution, as they are one of the leading causes of overdose for children and adults. An iron overdose can be deadly, so make sure you keep the iron out of reach of children. See the Iron Deficiency Overview chart for specific supplement information. Doses of 20 to 40 mg of elemental iron per day have been found to improve iron levels in people with anemia, but be sure to speak to your physician or pharmacist about a dose appropriate for you.

IRON DEFICIENCY OVERVIEW

Common Deficiency Causes	Acid-suppressing medications Heavy menses Blood loss Gut infections Food sensitivities Heavy metals
Optimal Levels	90–110 ng/mL
Supplement	Ferrochel from Designs for Health or OptiFerin-C from Pure Encapsulations
How to Take It	Please talk to your doctor or pharmacist for dosing guidelines. Take with vitamin C and betaine with pepsin.
Caution	Can be toxic and carries risk of overdose. Keep out of reach from children and pets.

Vitamin B_{12}

Low levels of B_{12} may lead to anemia, underdevelopment of villi (which house our digestive enzymes), impaired digestion, and inflammation. Vitamin B_{12} from our diet is found in animal proteins.

Lab tests for measuring B_{12} levels are available but do not always tell the whole story. Established "low" ranges are too low, and researchers have found that "normal-low" B_{12} levels have been associated with neurological symptoms such as difficulty balancing, memory lapses, brain fog, tingling of extremities, depression, mania, fatigue, and psychosis. Low levels of hydrochloric acid commonly found in those with Hashimoto's put people at risk for B_{12} deficiency. Intake of breads and cereals fortified with folic acid may mask this deficiency on standard lab tests.

Vitamin B_{12} is naturally found in animal products including fish, meat, poultry, eggs, milk, and other dairy products. However, this vitamin is generally not present in plant foods, which puts vegetarians and especially vegans at a greater risk for deficiency. Using a vitamin B_{12} supplement is essential for vegans and may be helpful for those with low stomach acid until the condition is corrected, as the B_{12} is in a free form and doesn't require separation.

Options for B_{12} replacement include tablets, sublinguals (under-the-tongue tablets), and injections. I prefer the sublingual route (as methylcobalamin) because it's better absorbed than the oral route and is more convenient than injections.

B_{12} DEFICIENCY OVERVIEW

Common Deficiency Causes	Vegan diet Vegetarian diet *H. pylori* infection Low stomach acid SIBO Acid blockers Gut disorders Weight-loss surgery
Optimal Levels	700–900 pg/mL
Supplement	B_{12} as methylcobalamin (Pure Encapsulations brand liquid or Designs for Health chewable)
How to Take It	5,000 mcg daily for 10 days, then 5,000 mcg weekly for 4 weeks, then 5,000 mcg monthly for maintenance
Caution	May cause irritability.

Additional Nutrient Tests

Some of my clients who choose to have SpectraCell's Micronutrient test—or as I like to call it, the Cadillac of nutrient testing—have shown additional deficiencies, especially in the following nutrients: selenium; all of the B vitamins, especially thiamine; fatty acids; zinc; glutathione; asparagine; oleic acid; inositol; and glutamine.

Another imbalance that may be seen in people with Hashimoto's is the MTHFR gene variation, whether homozygous (two copies of a mutated gene), heterozygous (one copy of a mutated gene), or compound heterozygous (one copy each of two different mutated genes). In the Liver Support Protocol, I recommended methylation support supplements for two weeks. These supplements will be important to take long-term if you have the MTHFR gene (see chapter 4).

For more information on self-order test options, please see sign up for the action plan at www.thyroidpharmacist.com/action.

Next Steps

I hope that going deeper into nutrition and nutrient strategies has helped reverse some of the Hashimoto's symptoms you long to be rid of. I know what it's like to need to keep digging—and the profound relief you feel when you discover a change that works. If any stubborn symptoms remain, do not despair, as there are more powerful steps for you to take in the other Advanced Protocols.

10

Protocols for Overcoming
Traumatic Stress

I f the traumatic stress assessment brought you here, let's look at some important next steps to help you heal from Hashimoto's. The Fundamental Adrenal Recovery Protocol combined with the Liver Support and Gut Balance Protocols can help repair many cases and types of adrenal dysfunction within the course of three months. But some people will continue to have adrenal dysfunction despite their best efforts to balance blood sugar and reduce present stressors. This is likely due to a long-standing history of traumatic stress that led to a deeply impaired stress response. Rebalancing the stress response in this case will take additional interventions. This includes taking inventory to address any traumatic stress that may be holding back your recovery and making sure your adrenals are being fully supported. Both of these are long-term strategies and should be done concurrently.

While working on the underlying psychological root causes of your impaired stress response, you may also find symptom relief by incorporating physiological adrenal-balancing therapies (beyond those you may have incorporated in the Adrenal Recovery Protocol). I generally recommend exploring both options. While you can get better with the tangible therapies (that is, supplements), there is a high likelihood of relapse into previous adrenal patterns if psychological vulnerabilities aren't addressed as well. Physical protocols will help you feel better in the short term, while the psychological ones will help you in the long term. This chapter will cover five psychological methods as well as advanced physical interventions that I've found to be helpful with my clients.

Creating an Anti-Inflammatory Environment, Inside and Out

In order to restore balance, we need to be sure that we are promoting an anti-inflammatory environment on all fronts. Inflammation is present in most autoimmune conditions and can trigger adrenal dysfunction as well as an autoimmune cascade. There may be a multitude of reasons for inflammation in the body, including infections, food intolerances, injuries, an imbalanced internal flora, and a pro-inflammatory environment created by an imbalanced omega-3 and omega-6 ratio. Furthermore, research shows that our thought patterns can be inflammatory. I see this thought-driven inflammation as a product of rumination.

Rumination is a term with multiple meanings; in psychology it refers to the act of reliving worries and stressors rather than focusing on solutions. When used to describe the eating patterns of animals, to ruminate means "to bring up and chew again what has already been chewed and swallowed." I like to draw a connection between these two meanings. In order to properly process difficult-to-digest foods, ruminant animals like cows and goats regurgitate and "rechew" the foods. This is a necessary process to ensure that the foods are properly digested; we know that undigested foods can be inflammatory, and this is a helpful process for the animals!

The same can be said about those difficult thoughts and experiences that are hard to assimilate, process, and "digest." Rather than digesting these thoughts and then moving on, people with an impaired stress response regurgitate these thoughts in their minds, which causes them distress. I'd like to add that though the rumination process is fine for ruminant animals, human beings are not cows or goats and have not evolved to thrive on rumination. Instead, rumination raises our inflammatory markers and worsens our adrenals. Though not widely known, there are helpful ways to process difficult-to-digest experiences. In this chapter, I will share with you some of the most helpful ways to overcome past traumas and stressors so that you can move on with your life and live a healthy and joyous existence free of intrusive, inflammatory thoughts.

In order to restore balance, we need to be sure that we are promoting an anti-inflammatory environment on all fronts.

Traumatic Stress and Hashimoto's

Early on in my journey with Hashimoto's, I didn't think much about the role that suppressed emotions and traumatic stress can play in autoimmune disease. But years of working with clients with underlying emotional trauma who failed to get well despite the best physical interventions opened my eyes (and mind) to the psychological component of Hashimoto's. When we think about the body as a system, this makes sense; just as our physical health can impact our mental health, the reverse is also true.

Stacey Robbins, a life coach who works specifically with women with Hashimoto's, has suggested that such traumatic events and emotional stress can be linked to behavior patterns often seen in women with Hashimoto's—patterns such as "perfectionism, control, mistrust, self-rejection, and fear-based living, just to name a few. It's a kickback response to unhealed situations in our past—whether it's sexual or physical abuse, or some kind of profound neglect, or a tragic event that occurred."

Do you recognize yourself in any of these patterns? If so, is it possible that underlying or unaddressed emotional trauma could be preventing you from healing completely? I know that even prying the box open to peer at something painful that you may have suppressed for years, even decades, is difficult. However, addressing events or experiences that may have shaped your heightened stress response or contributed to your thyroid dysfunction may be the missing link in creating complete healing from Hashimoto's. I know firsthand what it's like to look back at painful experiences, and I'd like to share a little with you about my own process if it can help encourage you to go further with yours.

Overcoming Traumatic Events and the Patterns They Lead To

Life traumas can put us into a fight-or-flight setting, but we can be reprogrammed with the right interventions. Having experienced trauma, abuse, and sexual assault may result in a person believing one or more of the following statements:

"The world is a dangerous place."
"People want to harm me."
"I am not safe here."
"I don't deserve to be loved."
"I need to protect myself."
"No one values me."
"No one will believe me."
"I am not enough."

In a way, these beliefs can serve a protective role in our lives. For example, a person who doesn't feel that the world is a safe place may become hypervigilant and more alert to potential threats, which could protect them from getting hurt. But these negative, self-limiting beliefs also lead to an obsession with control, feelings of being isolated and poorly understood, and always feeling at odds with the world around you. Furthermore, the negative experiences in our lives can lead us to form negative opinions of not just the world and people around us but also ourselves.

Root Cause Reflection: Do You Feel Safe?

Do you feel safe in your own home, community, body, and mind? This is a pretty deep question that goes beyond the usual health questionnaire I would give to my functional medicine clients when I first started consulting. Safety in my home, community, body, and mind was not something I considered for myself, or for others early in my journey, but I soon began to see a pattern, especially with the clients who, despite my (and their) best efforts, were not getting better.

Feeling unsafe keeps you from healing, as it put us in a fight-or-flight mode. As I mentioned in chapter 2, the thyroid gland can sense danger and initiate the autoimmune response. Many of my friends and readers know that I am a big evolution buff, so I can't help but wonder that perhaps our minds and bodies are sending a message to our thyroid and immune system in times we feel unsafe.

While I consider myself more practical than spiritual, this makes sense from a physiological standpoint nonetheless. Overactive fight-or-flight mode, which is a response of the sympathetic nervous system, is often present in people with a history of trauma and may predispose us to autoimmune disease—our emotions set our bodies to the fight-or-flight setting instead of the rest, digest, and heal setting.

I believe that Hashimoto's develops as a result of adaptive physiology. Your body wants to survive, and so it adapts to its environment. Hashimoto's becomes the body's defense mechanism for overwhelming stressors and threats. The threats could be toxins, infections, nutrient deficiencies, current stressful situations, or past unresolved emotional stressors. Hypothyroidism can play a protective role in the following cases:

- In cases of abuse, becoming hypothyroid makes us want to sleep and withdraw, where like the POWs, we have better chances of survival.
- In cases of sexual assault, hypothyroidism makes us less fertile and less attractive to potential abusers (hair loss, increased body weight, dull skin).
- The anxiety experienced due to thyroid cell breakdown may make a person more hypervigilant to potential dangers.

Research has connected physical and sexual abuse with excess weight gain later in life. It makes sense that someone who has had their physical or sexual boundaries violated would want to find ways to protect themselves. A person who was abused or felt vulnerable may feel protected by the excess weight. I believe that it's no coincidence that women are more likely to suffer both from sexual assault and autoimmune thyroid diseases.

In 2014, I attended a lecture by Erica Peirson, ND, who specializes in thyroid disorders in children with Down syndrome. She explained that more people in Ireland have Hashimoto's because the lower metabolic rate helped them survived the potato famine. Imagine that—thyroid disorders are advantageous in times of famine! This makes sense, as a person with a low metabolic rate can hold on to their body weight, fueling them when food is scarce. So if you're carrying around extra weight, thank your body for having this genius design, but also perhaps it's worth thinking about what may have convinced your body that you're going through a time of famine.

Here's the conversation that's happening inside of the body in times of stress. Immune system: "You're not safe here. This is not a good time to reproduce." Or "I'm going to help you get through the tough winter by slowing down your metabolism. This will allow you to hold on to more weight to keep you fed when food is scarce. I'm going to make you cold and tired so you don't venture out of your cave."

It may be easy for people to recognize environmental threats and physical abuse, but emotional abuse at the hands of others may also be a factor in you feeling unsafe. I know it can feel very hurtful and betraying when you realize that someone you love and trust is hurting you. But think about what your body is saying to you and why.

Alternatively, you may be someone who feels anxious, hypervigilant, and unsafe in response to normal life situations due to your past traumas. Furthermore, your own thought patterns may be contributing to your current state of stress.

I know it's not easy to make the first step toward change, but change is possible and you do not have to live this way. I don't know what kinds of traumas you have experienced in your life, but I can tell you that you are not alone and that your past does not determine your future. You can recover from your past, and you have the power to take back your health and your life! If you've suffered from severe trauma, you may want to seek treatment from a therapist. At the end of the chapter, I'll introduce you to the type of therapy I found most beneficial.

Do you feel safe?

Does thyroid disease play a protective role in your life?

From a philosophical standpoint, it's not a far stretch to connect negative self-beliefs to the immune system attacking our own body, but for all of you skeptical scientists like me, I'd like to share some research that supports the thyroid and emotional connection.

The first reported relationship between traumatic stress and autoimmune thyroid disease dates back to 1825, when a woman developed thyrotoxicosis shortly after her wheelchair was accidentally thrown down a flight of stairs. As early as 1927, Dr. Israel Bram reviewed three thousand cases of hyperthyroidism and found that significant traumatic stress had occurred in 85 percent of the cases before the onset of hyperthyroidism!

Most researchers long ago concluded that stress is a clear factor in the onset of Graves' disease. Because hyperthyroidism develops faster than hypothyroidism, it's easier to make this type of connection with Graves' than Hashimoto's. In contrast, Hashimoto's starts an average of ten years before most people are diagnosed. Nonetheless, most researchers have now concluded that traumatic stress can also be one of the environmental factors for developing Hashimoto's.

Research has connected childhood traumatic stress caused by physical abuse, sexual assault, neglect, home dysfunction, and the like to increased incidence of hospitalization due to autoimmune disease later in life. The link isn't limited to childhood; battered person syndrome, which is experienced by people who are victims of physical, emotional, and sexual abuse (usually at the hands of romantic partners), by definition includes health-related complaints such as asthma (an autoimmune disorder) and fibromyalgia (often connected to Hashimoto's).

In 2000, researchers Stein and Barrett-Connor found that past sexual assault was associated with an increased risk of breast cancer, arthritis, and thyroid disease. There are many more studies like this, including the following:

- Two additional studies found alterations in thyroid hormones in women who were sexually abused and had co-occurring menstrual-related mood disorders.
- Higher rates of Hashimoto's have also been found in victims of child abuse, with the researchers concluding, "Severe childhood trauma-related stress may promote lasting altered thyroid levels."
- A 1999 study by Wang and Mason reported that former prisoners of war (POWs) with evidence of combat-related post-traumatic stress disorder (PTSD) show decreased levels of free and total T3. These levels of thyroid hormone may be reflective of the ex-POWs' reports of "shutting-down" or "stonewalling," which were behaviors that were more life preserving compared to a fight-or-flight response, which may have put their lives in danger. Additional PTSD studies have found various alterations in thyroid hormone release patterns, such as higher levels of T4/T3 or lower levels of T4.
- Other studies have found that in nearly 80 percent of cases of autoimmune disease "patients reported uncommon emotional stress before disease onset."

Uncommon emotional stress has a wide-ranging definition—it suggests that everything from the loss of a loved one to a move or job change or new family addition could act as a trigger. These stressors can initiate or exacerbate an underlying autoimmune thyroid condition. Time and time again, my clients report that they began to feel unwell after one of the above-mentioned stressors.

Protocol for Resetting Your Stress Response

Most of us have a history of events that have somehow shaped us—this is part of being human. In some cases, our experiences have led to negative thoughts about ourselves and the world, which can in turn lead to the development of coping strategies and defense mechanisms. For example, as a result of various experiences in my own childhood,

How I Became Interested in the Autoimmune-Emotion Connection

Personally, I'm no stranger to traumatic events. Some of my traumas may feel insignificant compared to the suffering others have endured, but I can see how all of them together had a profound impact on my development.

The most significant traumatic event in my life was the unexpected death of a loved one in my early twenties. For me personally, my overt thyroid symptoms developed a few years after this loss, but I began to have hormonal alterations and eye floaters (flashes of lights in my peripheral vision that have been considered a possible symptom of thyroid cell breakdown) within days of the death.

A part of me thought that an experience like this was just a coincidence, but it turns out I wasn't alone in dealing with post-traumatic disease onset—20 percent of my readers with Hashimoto's reported that their symptoms started after the death of a loved one. I felt that in order to honor myself and others with the condition, I needed to properly process my traumas and bring them to the open so others wouldn't have to suffer alone.

Psychosomatic pain is a term used to describe pain that arises from psychological experiences and trauma, and therapists who specialize in somatic therapy report that traumas are stored within parts of our bodies. I remember having the worst ever neck pain on the day I found out this person had died. Later, I found that whenever I recalled this loss, my thyroid gland would ache and throb. I came to wonder if all of the pain I've ever experienced sat in my thyroid gland; it was as though my thyroid gland was a little locket that kept all of my pains and traumas inside of it, until the traumas became too big and painful to be contained and began to inflame the thyroid. Though I only noticed the pain when I focused on the trauma, I believe the inflammation was always there. The pain resolved when I was able to process the trauma through the therapy I will share later in this chapter. If you've gone through a traumatic event that you have not processed, perhaps a part of healing the thyroid gland is opening up to let the pain out.

I came to believe that the world was not a safe place, that I was not enough, and that I had to take care of myself. This led me to develop trust and control issues, extremely high standards for myself, and perfectionist and workaholic tendencies.

In a way, these coping mechanisms helped me get ahead in life. Thanks to my trust issues, very few people took advantage of me. My high expectations and workaholic and perfectionist tendencies helped me to graduate with my doctorate degree at age twenty-three and excel in numerous jobs. I found that the best way to get through sad situations was to go to work, keep myself busy, and achieve. I avoided idle time as much as possible, as being by myself and having extra time on my hands led me to being sad ... and so I developed these patterns that became cemented in my character.

The problem is, I didn't really know how to relax. I only had two settings: go and sleep. Even when my body started rejecting the all-nighters, the overcommitments, the caffeine, and the busy binges, I kept pushing on and I began to lose my health. In a way, you could say that my immune system attacking my thyroid was my body's way of slowing me down. When I was first diagnosed with Hashimoto's, I focused solely on fighting and addressing the physiological triggers to get myself well. I became a warrior, but when you're fighting an autoimmune disease, you are really fighting yourself.

While many of the physiologically driven lifestyle changes can certainly help people with healing their bodies, they do not address the underlying patterns that perpetuate the autoimmune response. After going into remission, many of my perfectionist and type A readers, who followed all of the dietary changes to a T, once again turned to the same patterns that got them sick in the first place (overextending, overworking, and people pleasing) despite the fact that they were following a gluten-free diet. This is why a holistic approach to Hashimoto's is so important.

It would be great if we could just tell our bodies, "Stop attacking yourself," right? And we can, but in order for this to be effective, we need to speak to our bodies in a way that it can understand that we are safe. How do you let your body know that you are safe? Treat your body as your cherished temple. Be nice to it by feeding it nutritious foods when it's hungry. Don't skip meals; don't subject it to unnecessary stresses like working all day instead of playing or resting. Sleep when you're tired. Don't cover it up with harsh makeup and skin creams. Stop forcing it to have more caffeine when you're tired. Let it rest. Don't drench it in antacids when it's trying to tell you a food you're eating is not working. Listen to it and care for it like you would care for a dear friend, pet, or child who's not feeling well.

The other critical part of ending the war within your body might come down to addressing some painful parts of your past and resetting your thought patterns about the world and about yourself. These were essential steps in my own healing, and they could be ones you also need to take before you can fully heal from Hashimoto's. I recommend that everyone start by completing the following steps. Start with the first four, and if you need additional help, look to the fifth step too.

Step 1: Practice Self-Love and Self-Kindness

People often want to be healed by others, but the healing really comes from within through the choices we make on a daily basis. One of the most important choices you can make is to choose to love yourself instead of choosing to attack yourself.

How do you show love to yourself? You can start with a hug. While I admit that hugging yourself sounds awkward and silly, I challenge you to try it. Right now. Wrap your arms around yourself and squeeze. You really can't help but smile.

There are other ways for you to show yourself some love. On a daily basis, ask yourself the question, "If I truly loved myself, what would I do?" If you're looking for suggestions, here is a list of some acts of self-compassion:

- Take a hot bath with no time limit.
- Get a massage.
- Buy yourself a special treat.
- Nourish yourself with great food.
- Say kind words to yourself.
- Speak your truth.
- Take a nap.
- Do something really nice for yourself.
- Ask for help when you need it.
- Talk to someone who will listen and not judge.

Step 2: Develop an Attitude of Gratitude

One of the fastest ways to feel better is to start a gratitude journal. Think of three things that you are grateful for each day and write them down in your journal. While you may be sick, there are still things you can be grateful for such as the food in your fridge, the funny things your kids say, the comfy pillows on your bed, that new great-smelling soap you just bought, the arms that let you carry your babies and hug the people you love ... just start with listing three things, no matter how big or small, each day and see how it makes you feel. I bet it's better and not worse.

When we are diagnosed with Hashimoto's, we can feel like our bodies are failing us, but maybe our bodies have a protective mechanism built in. This may sound cheesy, but I want you to try it. Instead of being angry and at war with your body, be grateful that your body is trying to help you survive and thank your body for letting you know that something is wrong.

Step 3: Seek Alpha Brain Waves

Shifting your brain into positive and relaxing thought patterns can help with reducing negative thought patterns and processing past traumas, or becoming "unstuck." Yoga and mindfulness practices, which I recommended in the Adrenal Recovery Protocol, can gently reshape your thought patterns. I also recommend the use of neurofeedback, a type of therapy that measures your brain waves and teaches you to have more positive thought patterns. These therapies are cumulative, meaning the more you do them, the better you'll feel.

Step 4: Find Support in Community

Having an invisible autoimmune condition can make a person feel completely and utterly alone. While friends and family members often rally around those with visible injuries or potentially terminal diagnoses like cancer, most are not gifted with the understanding of how to support a loved one with Hashimoto's. They may not understand your symptoms and may not understand why you are seeking treatments that go against the grain of conventional medicine to get yourself better. After all, chances are that you "don't look sick" to them. It's so important for you to know, as my friend Stacey Robbins says, "You're not crazy, and you're not alone!" Many others have gone through the same challenges you have had and can help support you through them. Whether that's a trusted friend, an online forum, a coach, or a therapist, find someone who will listen to you and be supportive.

Root Cause Research Corner: Social Stress

As human beings, we are wired to be social creatures. From an evolutionary standpoint, part of our survival depended on our ability to be connected socially within our communities. Thus feelings of defeat, disappointment, and social rejection may contribute to alterations of stress and thyroid hormones.

While studies in humans would be unethical, researchers have created controlled, socially stressful situations to test animals' hormonal responses to social stress. Scientists exposed male rats to simulated social defeat situations, where intruder rats were dropped into the cages of unfamiliar rat couples and subsequently attacked by the resident male rats, over and over. Four weeks of getting dropped into different rat cages and getting attacked by other rats left the intruder rats with altered thyroid hormones. T4 and T3 levels dropped by about 50 percent after one week of this social stress. Within four weeks, the rats started exhibiting behaviors that might reflect a loss of motivation (less exploring) and an inability to experience pleasure (not eating sugar, a favorite rat activity). In a related study, sheep isolated from their flocks were found to have altered thyroid hormone levels.

Having an autoimmune thyroid condition and even the lifestyle changes required to overcome the condition can feel isolating. The people that I continue to see struggling often lack social support and feel isolated, defeated, rejected, and unsupported.

I can't stress the importance of having a sense of community, support, and simply a person to talk to when you're going through your life, especially through your health journey. Time and time again, the people who do best are the ones who find support within the community, be it in person or online.

Step 5: Be Willing to Seek Deeper Treatments

Most people will benefit from yoga and meditation, journaling, and positive affirmations, but some will need to go beyond these exercises to resolve issues related to traumatic stress. If you are in this latter group, I recommend that you explore support groups, self-help books, emotional-freedom techniques, and even working with a specialized therapist to help you reshape your stress response.

There are several types of therapy, but because I prefer spending time on solutions and not dwelling as much on the past, I was particularly drawn to eye movement desensitization and reprocessing (EMDR) therapy. EMDR is a method used by psychotherapists to help people eliminate the lasting effect of traumatic events. This method can help people overcome traumatic events when other methods fail.

Francine Shapiro, PhD, an American psychologist and educator, initially developed this method after noticing that certain eye movements reduced the intensity of her disturbing thoughts and made her less anxious during a walk in nature. She tested the method with trauma victims and published her findings in 1989. The EMDR method was found equivalent in efficacy compared to trauma-focused cognitive behavior therapy and was found to be an evidence-based treatment for PTSD. I prefer EMDR because trauma-focused therapy can take a really long time and can make people feel worse before they feel better. An offshoot of EMDR known as induced after-death communication (IADC) can be especially helpful for processing traumas due to the loss of a loved one.

As the name may suggest, trauma-focused therapy centers on past traumas and opens up old wounds. Years of tears can surface like a faucet. In contrast, EMDR gives the brain a novel way to reprocess traumas without necessarily spending years digging into each one.

Although I spent close to a year in specialized grief therapy, and felt like it helped me a great deal, I still developed post-traumatic stress disorder after the loss of a loved one. Many years down the line,

Root Cause Reflection:
Change the Voice Inside Your Head

How many of us cut negative people out of our lives, say good-bye to unsupportive friends, minimize contact with mean relatives, and so on, but continue to beat ourselves up? I know I'm not alone in having been my own biggest hater and critic. These are some of the thoughts I used to direct toward myself:

"You're so dumb, I can't believe you said that in front of so-and-so."

"You're so awkward, people are going to laugh at you."

"You woke up late again? You're such a loser."

What I realized is that when I promised not to let anyone beat me up, "anyone" has to include me.

Let's reframe. Think of a time when you did something wrong. What did you say to yourself? Now imagine instead if this was your best friend, little sister, or daughter. Imagine she was tired from a long day of work and travel, then woke up late and missed two meetings. What would you say to her?

Chances are, you'd respond in a much more loving fashion. Instead of saying, "You fool! I can't believe you did that. You're failing at life." You'd likely say, "Sweetie, sorry to hear that you overslept and missed those important meetings. I'm sure you feel bad about it already. Maybe it's a sign that your body needs more rest. Maybe you've been working too hard. Be kind to yourself and take care of yourself."

The takeaway is that it's okay to be your own best friend. Treat yourself as gently and kindly as you would your little sister or your baby girl.

Who is that person in your life that you love unconditionally (a child, friend, family member, or perhaps even pet)?

What things do you say to yourself that you would never say to the person you love?

If you treated yourself like someone you truly loved unconditionally, what sorts of things would you say to yourself instead?

I still felt like the death had just happened, I often had nightmares, and I couldn't think or talk about the loss without feeling emotional or exhausted. I now realize that as I tried to suppress the trauma, it became toxic. EMDR helped me to properly process this significant trauma as well as other childhood traumas that are all too common in our world that led to my self-limiting thoughts and beliefs.

Though the number of sessions you will need will ultimately be determined by the number of past traumatic events you have had, EMDR can begin to produce results within a single session. It successfully allows patients to become desensitized to previously devastating traumas! I now can separate the difference between what happened and what I made it mean, which had been a challenge for me before.

Advanced Adrenal Support Protocol

Resetting our stress response is a journey. I recommend a two-pronged approach, addressing both the psychology and the physiology behind your stress response dysfunction. Now that you have an action plan for addressing your past, let's talk about addressing your stress hormones in the present time.

Normal-functioning adrenals produce cortisol in a rhythm. A cortisol kick in the morning helps us to get out of bed bright-eyed and bushy-tailed, ready to face the day, and then lessened cortisol

Root Cause Reflection: A Journey Through Trauma

Have you experienced traumas in your life that led you to develop negative beliefs about the world?

Do any of these traumas affect your health, well-being, or happiness?

What will happen if you don't overcome your traumas?

What is your plan for overcoming these traumas in your life?

"Today I choose to love me. Today I choose to cherish me. I will no longer attack myself, beat myself up, or be hard on myself. I deserve better. I deserve love, compassion, caring, and understanding. I will not settle for less. Today it starts with me."

secretion at bedtime helps us relax and sleep. Some people with adrenal dysfunction have a flipped cortisol rhythm, where their adrenals put out very little cortisol in the morning and too much in the evening, causing them to be alert and sleepy at the wrong times.

Other people may have abnormally low cortisol readings all day, every day. These people will wake up tired and feel fatigued all day (this was me—it's not fun). Low cortisol can also cause inflammation to go unchecked in the body and prevent healing.

It's possible to reset this rhythm through the use of supplements. Using licorice root drops in the morning (not deglycyrrhizinated licorice, or DGL) can help boost low cortisol readings through extending the life of cortisol in the body, while using phosphatidylserine at bedtime can reduce cortisol. You can also balance out cortisol production with pregnenolone and dehydroepiandrosterone (DHEA) over-the-counter hormonal supplements. For underperforming adrenals, adrenal glandulars as well as the medication hydrocortisone may be helpful.

Although most of these hormones are available over the counter at health food stores, they are certainly not benign and should be used under the supervision of a trained professional with extreme caution. Pregnenolone and DHEA are hormone and steroid precursors, and can potentially fuel hormone-dependent tumors, while licorice can exacerbate high blood pressure. Hydrocortisone can cause weight gain and hypothalamic-pituitary-adrenal (HPA) axis suppression when used in high doses or for prolonged periods. It's important to work with a practitioner who is knowledgeable about the use of these hormones.

Before trying these, it's important that you first get a test for adrenal dysfunction. This is because treatment for each stage of adrenal dysfunction requires a different combination of the above-mentioned supplements, in varying doses.

I recommend the salivary Functional Adrenal Stress Profiles test from BioHealth Laboratory as well as the DUTCH adrenal hormone panel, which I have found to be the most accurate for adrenal testing. For recommended brands of supplements, please go to www.thyroid pharmacist.com/action.

Adrenal Saliva Test Results

While I shared some of the symptoms associated with the different stages of adrenal dysfunction in chapter 5, and these may guide you to "guesstimate" the level of adrenal dysfunction you may have, for the purposes of using hormones, I recommend getting an adrenal saliva test to determine your precise stage of adrenal dysfunction and working with a practitioner who is trained to administer these hormones.

Adrenal saliva results will measure four cortisol readings throughout the day (morning, noon, afternoon, and bedtime) and will also add up the day's total cortisol. Cortisol is a hormone that gives us an energy kick. Healthy adrenal rhythms will start off with high morning cortisol so that we can be bright-eyed and bushy-tailed and ready to take on the day, and then the cortisol readings get progressively lower throughout the day.

At bedtime, cortisol should be at its lowest so we can get the rest we need. Alternations in the four cortisol readings are key to how a person is feeling throughout the day. For example, a person with a low morning cortisol will likely have a hard time waking up in the morning and feel sluggish, while a person with high bedtime cortisol will have trouble falling asleep. A person who has increased cortisol readings as the day progresses will likely feel anxious or irritable around the times of those readings.

After reviewing hundreds of adrenal saliva tests with Hashimoto's clients, I'm amazed at their ability to accurately portray how a person feels.

The protocols I'm listing below have helped my clients recover their adrenal function, when used for a period of three months to two years.

Pregnenolone and DHEA are dosed two to three times per day in every stage of adrenal dysfunction, while licorice root is only utilized before low cortisol readings to help stretch cortisol, while Phosphatidyl Serine is only utilized before high cortisol readings to help with clearing cortisol from the body.

Adrenal Hormonal Protocols per Saliva Test Results

Stage 1: High-cortisol stage: In this initial stage, the HPA axis is overresponsive. An adrenal saliva test would reveal high total cortisol and borderline, low, or normal DHEA. Protocol:

* Pregnenolone: 6–8 mg, 2–3 times per day for 3–6 months
* DHEA: 4 mg, 2–3 times per day for 3–6 months
* Phosphatidyl Serine (soy free) by ProThera: Take 30 minutes prior to high cortisol reading for 1–2 weeks

Stage 2: Cortisol-dominant stage: Now DHEA is either low or borderline, and overall cortisol levels are normal, but an adrenal saliva test may reveal fluctuations in the cortisol rhythm, such as excessively high cortisol in the morning but lowered later in the day. As this continues, the adrenals eventually become exhausted and start to burn out, progressing to the third stage. Protocol:

- Pregnenolone: 8–12 mg, 2–3 times per day for 3–12 months
- DHEA: 2–3 mg, 2–3 times per day for 3–12 months
- Phosphatidyl Serine (soy free) by ProThera: Take 2–4 hours prior to high cortisol reading for 1–2 weeks

Stage 3: Low-cortisol stage: In this stage, DHEA is either low or borderline low, and the total cortisol is low. Protocol:

- Pregnenolone: 10–15 mg, 2–3 times per day for 3 months to 2 years
- DHEA: 1–3 mg, 2–3 times per day for 3 months to 2 years
- Hydrocortisone: 5–15 mg per day in divided doses, if total cortisol is under 15 nM/L, for 1 to 6 months
- Licorice drops: 5–10 drops taken 4 hours prior to low cortisol readings for 3–6 months (do not use with high blood pressure)

Cautions: While most of the supplements I recommend in this book are generally well tolerated and highly unlikely to cause adverse reactions, the hormonal protocol supplements are an exception to this. All of the above-listed supplements have the propensity to impact hormone levels, and while they are available without a prescription, I do recommend that they be used only under the supervision of a trained practitioner.

Pregnenolone: Not to be taken with history of hormone-dependent cancers or tumors or with hyperthyroidism. Do not start with full dose at once.

> ## Additional Adrenal Resources
>
> For further reading on adrenals, you can check out my other book, *Hashimoto's Thyroiditis: Lifestyle Interventions for Finding and Treating the Root Cause*, or any of these excellent resources:
>
> - *The Adrenal Reset Diet* by Alan Christianson
> - *Adrenal Fatigue* by James L. Wilson
> - *The Adrenal Thyroid Revolution* by Aviva Romm

DHEA: Not to be taken with history of hormone-dependent cancers, tumors, estrogen dominance, high DHEA, high testosterone, hyperthyroid, or polycystic ovary syndrome (PCOS). Do not start with full dose at once. Excess dose may cause acne; in that case, reduce dose or discontinue.

Hydrocortisone: Numerous possible precautions and side effects, including pituitary and adrenal suppression when used in excess. May suppress the immune system and encourage the spread of low-grade infections.

Licorice drops: Do not take with high blood pressure. Will increase blood pressure.

Phosphatidyl Serine: Do not take with stage 3 adrenal fatigue, reduced kidney function, or caffeine.

Adrenal Glandulars

Depending on the origin of adrenal dysfunction, adrenal glandulars or sometimes pituitary or hypothalamic glandulars may be utilized in conjunction with, or in place of, the above protocols to help support the production of adrenal hormones. Some brands of quality glandulars include Standard Process, Biotics Research, and Allergy Research Group.

Next Steps

As we have just covered, trauma and stress play a major role in both the development of Hashimoto's and the way in which it can radically alter your symptoms. Hopefully this Advanced Protocol helped to clarify this connection and provided you with the guidance you needed to help alleviate your symptoms. I know I feel much better having shared this very vital and at times very personal information with you. Remember that the practice of compassionate self-care is a long-term strategy for your best health. Be kind to you, always.

11

Protocols for Addressing Infections

C hronic infections are the Hashimoto's triggers that get the least amount of attention, yet identifying and treating them can result in complete remission of Hashimoto's. It's important to pay attention to infections because some of them can be progressive and lead to an increasing number of symptoms if they're not identified and treated accordingly.

This chapter will cover testing for chronic infections, infection-specific protocols for the most common infections found in people with Hashimoto's, as well as a broad-spectrum infection protocol that can be used in the absence of positive test results.

You might wonder where these infections can hide in your body. The truth is, they can live anywhere, such as in your gums, sinuses, thyroid gland, and gut. These infections can contribute to the development of autoimmunity through various mechanisms, depending on where they live: molecular mimicry, if outside the thyroid gland, and the bystander effect or thyroid-directed autoimmunity, if inside the thyroid gland (see chapter 2 for more on this). The infections that live in the gut, gums, or sinuses can also contribute directly to intestinal permeability.

Scientists have found a great deal of evidence that suggests that Hashimoto's is caused by infections. Hashimoto's patients often have positive blood tests indicating a past or current exposure to

Root Cause Research Corner: Debunking the Hygiene Hypothesis in Hashimoto's

We know that autoimmune disease tends to be more common in places with higher socioeconomic status; this has led to the development of the hygiene hypothesis of autoimmunity. This theory suggests that the reason we get autoimmune disease is because we are too clean and don't have enough infections during childhood, leading to a poorly developed immune system. This immune response has been compared to a bored police officer in a small town who, instead of looking for criminals, begins to harass good citizens for minor offenses. Some will use this theory as an argument against treating infections in Hashimoto's, suggesting that infections help promote immune system balance.

However, while the hygiene hypothesis has received some scientific validation related to other diseases, it has not proven relevant in Hashimoto's. One study found that rodents raised in a germ-free environment were at greater risk for type 1 diabetes, but this same effect was not seen in Hashimoto's. In fact, rodents raised under conventional conditions developed thyroiditis more commonly than rodents in pathogen-free conditions. A 2016 study revealed that Hashimoto's, asthma, and rheumatoid arthritis were still present in similar amounts in a rural Peruvian village with a high prevalence of parasitic infections compared to industrialized countries. Thus infections have not been found to help prevent autoimmune conditions but may instead make them worse. If you are found to have an infection, I recommend treating it accordingly.

an infection, and many patients can trace the onset of their condition to a bout of illness. However, scientists have yet to say that Hashimoto's is caused by infection because they're looking for that one single infection in every person with Hashimoto's. But it's not a black-and-white thing. It's too simplistic to think that an infection can only be a root cause if every person with the disease has it and every person without the disease does not. In my observation, the equation is more complex. It's more likely to be a combination of factors: genes combined with infection A and perhaps infection B, C, and even D, coupled with the absence of nutrients and beneficial bacteria can lead to the development of an autoimmune condition.

Numerous infectious pathogens can have protein sequences similar to the thyroid gland, numerous infections have the ability to infect the thyroid gland, and many types of infections can cause leaky gut. Some new research even suggests that even our friendly bacteria (*Lactobacillus* species) has a similar protein sequence to the thyroid gland, so in the case of leaky gut, the good bacteria can get into our bloodstream and cause an immune response, which can potentially cross-react with thyroid tissue.

All of those scenarios are potential mechanisms for how various infections could lead to developing autoimmune disease.

The Many Infections Linked to Hashimoto's

Many infections have been implicated in triggering and exacerbating Hashimoto's. Here's a partial list of infections that I have seen in clients or that have been reported in research:

- *Bartonella henselae,* "cat scratch fever"
- *Blastocystis hominis*
- *Borrelia burgdorferi,* the bacteria that causes Lyme
- Coxsackie virus
- *Cryptosporidium*
- Cytomegalovirus

- *Dientamoeba fragilis*
- *Endolimax nana*
- *Entamoeba histolytica*
- Enterovirus
- Erythrovirus B19
- *Giardia lamblia*
- *H. pylori*
- Hepatitis C
- Herpes viruses
- Human herpesvirus 6
- Human parvovirus
- Human T-lymphotropic virus type 1 (HTLV-1)
- *Iodamoeba bütschlii*
- Mumps
- *Mycobacterium avium subspecies paratuberculosis*
- Rubella
- Sinus infections
- Small intestinal bacterial overgrowth (SIBO)
- *Toxoplasma gondii*
- *Yersinia enterocolitica*

If you have Hashimoto's and you've had difficulty going into remission, there is a significant chance that you have an infection. Up to 80 percent of my clients who don't go into remission with dietary changes have tested for one or more infections using functional medicine testing. As we used to say in pharmacology class, "every bug needs a different drug," meaning that each infection has a unique treatment protocol. I'd like to share the top tests I recommend to clients to figure out if they have one or more of the above infections so that they can follow the appropriate protocols. Please note that no tests are perfect and that false negatives may also be present. That said, there are no false positives

While numerous infections have been implicated in triggering Hashimoto's, the most common infections I see in my clients include

SIBO, *H. pylori,* yeast overgrowth, *Blastocystis hominis,* and reactivated Epstein-Barr virus, so we will focus on these infections here.

Testing for Infections

- **H. pylori:** I recommend using the stool antigen test for *H. pylori,* which is a more sensitive test compared to an *H. pylori* breath test and even an endoscopy. Unlike the blood test, which may be positive due to past infections, a positive stool antigen test will reveal if a current infection is present. In 2015, 20 percent of my clients tested positive to *H. pylori.* Labs that utilize the stool antigen test include the BioHealth Lab 401/401H test, the GI-MAP test from Diagnostic Solutions Laboratory, the Doctor's Data Comprehensive Stool Analysis, the GI Pathogen Plus Profile from DRG Laboratory, and the GI Effects Comprehensive Profile—Stool from Genova Diagnostics.

- **Blastocystis hominis:** This protozoal parasite is the most common parasite I've found in people with Hashimoto's. In 2015, 35 percent of my clients tested positive for it. Functional medicine stool tests that test for this include the BioHealth Lab 401/401H test, the GI-MAP test from Diagnostic Solutions Laboratory, the Doctor's Data Comprehensive Stool Analysis, the GI Pathogen Plus Profile from DRG Laboratory, and the GI Effects Comprehensive Profile—Stool from Genova Diagnostics.

- **Yeast overgrowth:** Yeast overgrowth can be detected on stool tests like the BioHealth 401/401H test, the GI-MAP test from Diagnostic Solutions Laboratory, the Doctor's Data Comprehensive Stool Analysis, the GI Pathogen Plus Profile from DRG Laboratory, and the GI Effects Comprehensive Profile—Stool from Genova Diagnostics as well as organic acids tests offered by various labs.

- **SIBO:** A 2007 study revealed that SIBO can be present in up to 54 percent of people with hypothyroidism. Unfortunately, most stool tests do not test for the presence of SIBO. To properly test for SIBO, we need to do a breath test to determine the presence of gas-producing bacteria. Some gastroenterology centers may have breath-testing machines; otherwise, you can order a SIBO breath test kit that uses Lactulose to stimulate the bacteria to release their giveaway gases. SIBO breath tests are offered by the following labs: Commonwealth Laboratories, BioHealth Laboratory, and Genova Diagnostics.

- **Epstein-Barr virus reactivation:** Most of us have had a prior infection of the Epstein-Barr virus. In some, the virus may not be properly suppressed and may cause or exacerbate autoimmune disease. Blood tests are used to figure out if a person has a reactivated infection. Here's what to test (I recommend testing for all three, as only one may come out positive), and what the results may mean:

  - EBV-VCA IgG/IgM by ELISA (viral capsid antigen): IgG positive means you've had or have the infection; IgM positive means reactivated infection.
  - EBV-EBNA-1 IgG by ELISA (nuclear antigen): A positive test result is usually associated with past infection.
  - EBV-EA-D IgG by ELISA (early antigen): Positive EA IgG may mean active infection or reactivated infection.

Gut Infections in Hashimoto's: Overview and Recommended Protocols

Here are the most common gut infections I see in my Hashimoto's clients and protocols for addressing each infection. For all of the infections, I've listed pharmacological, herbal, and supportive protocols. In general, the prescription protocols are going to be more aggressive in nature, shorter lasting, and associated with more side effects. In contrast, the herbal protocols will usually be gentler, better tolerated, and longer lasting. In many cases, the herbal protocols can be used as an alternative to medication protocols or can be used before or after medication protocols. The supportive protocols are meant to be complementary protocols that can be used in conjunction with the medication or herbal protocols to accelerate healing, but they are not likely to suppress infections on their own accord. The risks and benefits of each treatment option should be discussed with your practitioner, and therapies should be tailored based on your history, symptoms, and goals. I recommend working with a knowledgeable practitioner to help you determine the best protocol for you.

H. Pylori

H. pylori is a gram-negative spirochete-shaped bacterium that burrows into our stomach lining and secretes urease, which neutralizes stomach acid. The by-product of the urease and stomach acid is toxic to epithelial cells, as are the other chemicals produced by this bacterium, leading to damage to cells, a disruption of tight junctions, and inflammation.

This bacterium can trigger an immune response and has been implicated in numerous autoimmune conditions, including Hashimoto's. While *H. pylori* is thought to be common in asymptomatic individuals—it can affect as many as 50 percent of people worldwide—I believe that, similar to all autoimmune triggers, *H. pylori* is part of the perfect storm in a genetically susceptible and vulnerable individual.

H. pylori has been implicated in ulcers and can contribute to low stomach acid, leading people to improperly digest their foods. In turn, the poorly digested foods are not broken down properly, and thus the person ends up with multiple food sensitivities as a result of this infection. Only a small percentage, perhaps 5 to 10 percent of those infected with *H. pylori*, will develop an ulcer. Others may have acid reflux.

H. pylori is transmitted orally from person to person as well as potentially between people and their pets (who can resist doggy kisses, right?).

H. Pylori *Protocol*

Here are some potential treatment options to discuss with your practitioner. While the treatment will depend on you and your practitioner, some patients prefer the longer, more gentle approach for asymptomatic cases and the more intensive and shorter approach in cases with symptoms.

PHARMACOLOGIC TREATMENT

The following medication treatments are considered the standard of care options for treating *H. pylori* infections.

Triple therapy:

- Omeprazole, amoxicillin, and clarithromycin (OAC) for 10 days
- Bismuth subsalicylate, metronidazole, and tetracycline (BMT) for 14 days
- Lansoprazole, amoxicillin, and clarithromycin (LAC), which has been approved for either 10 days or 14 days of treatment

Quadruple therapy:

- PPI, bismuth, tetracycline, and metronidazole for 7–14 days

HERBAL AND ALTERNATIVE TREATMENT

- Mastic gum: 500 mg, 2–3 times per day (breakfast, lunch, dinner) for 60 days
- DGL Plus: 1 tablet, 3 times per day (breakfast, lunch, dinner) for 60 days
- *S. boulardii:* 5 billion–15 billion CFUs, 2–4 times per day for 60 days (Please note, the use of multiple antibiotics has been implicated with dysbiosis and exacerbating gut issues. Taking *S. boulardii* along with antibiotic treatments may minimize the risk of dysbiosis.)

SUPPORTIVE TREATMENT

- Cabbage juice: 4 oz. daily for 28 days

Blastocystis Hominis

By far the most common parasite I've found in people with Hashimoto's is *Blastocystis hominis*. Many conventional physicians have regarded this parasite as a commensal organism and will say that there is no need to treat it, but multiple studies have implicated it in IBS and hives. These two conditions are very commonly associated with Hashimoto's. I personally had a *Blastocystis hominis* infection that had to be resolved before I felt completely well.

Symptoms of *Blastocystis hominis* can include bloating, diarrhea, nausea, flatulence, variable bowel habits, abdominal pain, hives, and fatigue. Additionally, this pathogen is notorious for causing multiple food sensitivities. A true food sensitivity, like celiac disease, usually results in a resolution of symptoms once food is removed, but *Blastocystis hominis*–infected people will have multiple food sensitivities and will keep getting more. For me personally, once I eradicated *Blastocystis hominis*, I began to tolerate foods that I previously did not tolerate, including grains, dairy, and eggs. Clients have experienced a similar outcome, reporting a reduction in food sensitivities, pain, fatigue, and thyroid antibodies. In research archives, a 2015 published case report described how eradication on *Blastocystis hominis* resulted in a normalization of thyroid function and a reduction of thyroid antibodies.

Often, *Blastocystis* co-occurs with *H. pylori,* and some professionals will go as far as to treat a person for both infections when one or the other is found.

Blastocystis Hominis *Protocol*

PHARMACOLOGIC TREATMENT

- Alinia: 1,000 mg twice a day for 3 days, repeated in 2 weeks, then again 2 weeks later
- Alternative options: Alinia 500 mg twice daily for 30 days, or Alinia 1,000 mg twice per day for 2 weeks (but Alinia will kill off lots of good flora and you may have extreme

die-off symptoms including exhaustion, body pains, and mood changes)

- Nystatin 500,000 units: 2 capsules, 3 times per day for 30–90 days with Alinia or after treatment to address the fungal overgrowth

HERBAL AND ALTERNATIVE TREATMENT

- CandiBactin-BR: 2 capsules, 3 times per day for 60 days
- Oil of oregano 150 mg: 2 capsules, 3 times per day for 60 days
- *S. boulardii:* 5 billion–15 billion CFUs, 2–4 times per day (up to 8 per day) for 60 days
- Wormwood-containing antiparasitic: 600 mg, 2 times per day for 7 days, repeat in 2 weeks (Do not use if you have a history of hepatitis or elevated liver enzymes.)

SUPPORTIVE TREATMENT

- Root Cause Paleo or Root Cause Autoimmune Diet for 90 days
- Lipase-containing digestive enzyme (Digestive Enzymes Ultra from Pure Encapsulations): As needed with meals for 60–90 days

Yeast Overgrowth

Yeast is an opportunistic organism that acts up when your overall health is impaired or when your immune system is compromised. Most people with Hashimoto's will have a high degree of yeast overgrowth, especially of the *Candida* genus. Treating this overgrowth can be very helpful in restoring health.

A note about *Candida: Candida* can be a primary or a secondary root cause. While conventional medicine underdiagnoses issues related to yeast overgrowth, natural medicine practitioners seem to overdiagnose yeast and may say *Candida* is a root cause for all ailments. I recommend a *Candida* protocol for most people with Hashimoto's, but if you have already done a similar protocol and found that it only worked temporarily (whether recurring through reemerging symptoms or on tests), you should consider that you may have a different underlying root cause. The following potential root causes can lead to a yeast overgrowth or can mimic the symptoms of a yeast infection:

- Parasitic infection
- Dysbiosis
- Heavy metal toxicity: yeast overgrows whenever there are heavy metals present
- SIBO

Yeast Overgrowth Protocol

PHARMACOLOGIC TREATMENT

- Nystatin 500,000 units: 2 capsules, 3 times per day for 30–90 days (Diflucan is an alternative option)

HERBAL AND ALTERNATIVE TREATMENT

- Oil of oregano 150 mg: 2 capsules, 3 times per day for 60 days
- *S. boulardii:* 5 billion–15 billion CFUs, 2–4 times per day (up to 8 per day) for 60 days
- Activated charcoal: 2–4 capsules daily at bedtime for 60 days (may deplete magnesium)

SUPPORTIVE TREATMENT

- Anti-yeast diet, such as the Body Ecology Diet, for 60–90 days

SIBO

SIBO is an overgrowth of bacteria in the small intestine. Generally, the small intestine is supposed to have less bacteria than the colon, but in some cases more bacteria may get into the small intestine and promote intestinal permeability as the body tries to get rid of the bacteria. This overgrowth can be caused by a variety of issues such as low stomach acid, antibiotic use, acid-suppressing medication use, slowed GI transit, and food poisoning, among others.

SIBO can lead to many digestive symptoms like bloating, acid reflux, belching, and irritable bowel syndrome (diarrhea, constipation, or mixed type) and can cause a depletion of vitamin B_{12} and iron. Furthermore, SIBO leads to the destruction of many digestive enzymes like lactase (digests lactose in dairy) and amylase (digests starch), making it more difficult to digest many foods.

SIBO Protocol

PHARMACOLOGIC TREATMENT

- For hydrogen-producing bacteria: Rifaximin 1,200 mg daily for 14 days
- For methane-producing bacteria: Rifaximin 1,600 mg per day for 10 days, combined with neomycin (1,000 mg daily for 10 days) or metronidazole (750 mg per day for 10 days)

HERBAL AND ALTERNATIVE TREATMENT

- CandiBactin-BR: 2 capsules, 3 times per day for 60 days
- Oil of oregano 150 mg: 2 capsules, 3 times per day for 60 days
- For methane-producing bacteria, add Allicillin (garlic extract): 2 capsules, 3 times per day for 60 days

SUPPORTIVE TREATMENT

- Peppermint tea: 2–3 cups per day
- Physicians' Elemental Diet by Integrative Therapeutics used as meal replacement for 2–3 weeks (may exacerbate adrenal issues)
- Specific carbohydrate diet for 60–90 days
- GAPS diet for 60–90 days
- Low-FODMAP diet for 60–90 days

An Important Note on Diets for Infections

While I have listed supportive diets for most of the infections common to Hashimoto's, please keep in mind that many of these infections cannot be treated by diet alone. People can improve their symptoms by diet, but by no means will that fully heal the infections, with the exception of perhaps SIBO, which can be eradicated through following an elemental diet over the course of two to three weeks. So be sure to work with your practitioner to get a comprehensive treatment!

Retesting

To ensure that the SIBO has indeed been eradicated and not just reduced, it's important to retest with another breath test within two weeks of finishing SIBO treatment.

In some cases, a person may have regrowth of SIBO due to low stomach acid, valve abnormalities, or poor GI motility. In these cases, prophylactic use of betaine with pepsin for stomach acid support and prophylactic use of prokinetic agents that aid in GI motility, such as low-dose naltrexone, low-dose erythromycin, *Lactobacillus rhamnosus,* and *Bifidobacterium lactis* probiotics, and the German herbal blend Iberogast, may help to prevent recurrences.

Broad-Spectrum Gut Infection

In the event that you would prefer not to test for gut infections or your test results were negative, you can also try the broad-spectrum natural protocol to help support your body in fighting off gut infections. For best results, make sure that you're supporting your detox pathways and your adrenals during the gut-cleansing protocol introduced here.

While this more general gut cleanse will help some individuals eradicate gut pathogens, eliminate some parasites, and improve or remove SIBO, dysbiosis, and yeast overgrowth, not everyone will be successful by following this alone. Certainly, doing a general gut cleanse is better than doing nothing, but a more specific protocol might be needed simply because different bugs are sensitive to different drugs (and herbs).

The broad-spectrum natural protocol has activity against various pathogens and may be helpful in balancing your gut flora.

If you have elevated thyroid antibodies, it may help to remeasure them after the broad-spectrum protocol to make sure you are on the right track.

Root Cause Broad-Spectrum Gut-Cleansing Protocol

- Oil of oregano 150 mg: 2 capsules, 3 times per day for 60 days
- CandiBactin-BR: 2 capsules, 3 times per day for 60 days
- *S. boulardii:* 5 billion–15 billion CFUs, 2–4 times per day (up to 8 per day) for 60 days
- Wormwood-containing antiparasitic: 600 mg, 2 times per day for 7 days, repeat in 2 weeks (Do not use if you have a history of hepatitis or elevated liver enzymes.)

Looking Beyond Gut Infections

Functional medicine has taught us that the gut is at the center of autoimmune disease. However, remember that intestinal permeability can be caused not just by infections that live in the gut but also by infections in the gums and sinuses, and throughout the body. Here, I'll introduce you to the most common infections outside the gut that can complicate healing in Hashimoto's. Each of these may require seeking the assistance of a specialist to diagnose and treat. I recommend working with a biological dentist to screen for infections in the mouth as well as receiving an evaluation for sinus infections.

Periodontitis

Periodontitis is an inflammation of the gums that can lead to the receding of the gums, loose teeth, and eventually tooth loss. Symptoms may include bleeding gums (especially with brushing or flossing), puffy gums, receding gums, plaque buildup on teeth, loose teeth, bone loss in the jaw, and bad breath. Periodontitis is often found in Hashimoto's patients and can be worsened by fluoride, the very substance added to our waters and toothpastes to prevent tooth decay.

Pathogens that cause periodontitis have been suggested to contribute to rheumatoid arthritis and Hashimoto's through molecular mimicry.

While previous research implicated oral bacteria in triggering periodontitis, French-Canadian dentist Dr. Mark Bonner has found that most cases of periodontitis are caused by two parasitic infections of the gums: *Entamoeba gingivalis* and *Trichomonas tenax*. *Entamoeba gingivalis* was found in 69 percent of diseased gingival pockets but was absent in healthy gum tissue. This bug is transferred from person to person through kissing and may also be present in dogs, cats, and horses. The parasite *Trichomonas tenax* may be found in another 5 to 20 percent of cases of periodontitis and is also found in people, cats, and dogs.

If you have these symptoms or suspect you might have periodontitis or another type of infection in your mouth, I recommend working with a biological dentist in your area and requesting an infection screening.

Treatments for Periodontitis

Advanced cases of periodontitis will require dental interventions, including anti-infective medications and specialized dental cleaning of the gums. Antiprotozoal agents with activity against amoebas such as metronidazole, nitazoxanide (Alinia), and the Root Cause Broad-Spectrum Gut-Cleansing Protocol may be helpful in suppressing the pathogens due to their amoebicidal activity, but they may not be able to penetrate the gingival pockets deeply enough to get to all of the organisms.

If you continue to have periodontitis after undergoing treatments with antiprotozoal medications or herbs, or if the periodontitis comes back after a few months, you may require additional dental interventions. As this amoeba is passed through person-to-person kissing, you may also want to make sure your kissing partners are treated accordingly.

Dr. Bonner has created a protocol that involves the use of pharmaceuticals (antiparasitics, antifungals, antibiotics) and advanced dental cleaning methods and testing of the periodontal pockets to ensure eradication of *Entamoeba gingivalis* and *Trichomonas tenax* and a return of healthy gum flora. He reports that this method is a cure for periodontitis and has trained over six hundred dentists on the method. For more information on Dr. Bonner's protocol and additional dental guidance, I recommend his book *To Kiss or Not to Kiss* and the website www.parodontite.com.

Suppressive Treatments for Periodontitis

In some cases, suppressive treatments for periodontitis may be helpful in managing the symptoms. The antibiotic doxycycline has become the drug of choice for many cases of periodontitis, as it has greater availability in the gingival crevice compared to other medications. It penetrates the gums seven to twenty times more effectively than other drugs. Interestingly, this same antibiotic has been reported to eliminate TPO antibodies for some, perhaps through the suppression of periodontitis or the "food source" of another pathogen, and may be an option to consider in people with both Hashimoto's and periodontitis.

Doxycycline works in three helpful ways for periodontitis (these are examples of prescription protocols that might be prescribed by a dentist):

- **Antimicrobial activity against various mouth pathogens implicated in periodontics:** The recommended antimicrobial dose of doxycycline is 100 mg twice per day on the first day, followed with 100 mg once daily for twenty-one days.

- **Downregulation of the enzymes that lead to gum destruction:** Subantimicrobial doses of this drug, considered to be too low to treat bacteria, can still be effective for reducing periodontitis. As an adjunctive treatment for periodontitis, take 20 mg twice daily for up to nine months.
- **Prevention of bone loss in the jaw:** Doxycycline can slow bone loss from periodontitis. However, eradication protocols can reverse it!

Natural and Complementary Suppressive Approaches

Tactics that may be helpful for displacing the pathogenic bacteria from teeth and reducing the inflammation associated with periodontitis that may be contributing to Hashimoto's include changing your diet to a Root Cause type diet, proper tooth brushing, eliminating pathogenic mouth bacteria, and following the Root Cause Basic Dental Protocol. We've already covered the various diets, so let's take a closer look at tooth brushing, eliminating bacteria, and the protocol.

PROPER TOOTH BRUSHING

Many of us are not familiar with proper brushing techniques. While brushing your teeth, aim at the gum line, as that's where most of the pathogenic bacteria live. You can do this by angling your toothbrush up to reach upper gums, and angling it down to reach lower gums.

The most helpful way to brush is through applying gentle pressure and a jiggling motion; sonic toothbrushes can do the work for you. Flossing is also an important daily habit. This will help to dislodge food particles (aka food for pathogenic bacteria).

ELIMINATING PATHOGENIC MOUTH BACTERIA

Eliminating pathogenic mouth bacteria can be challenging, as the mouth bacteria form biofilms, also known as dental plaques, that protect them from the usual methods of removal. These are some strategies that may help eliminate bacteria:

- **Waterpikking:** Using a Waterpik may be helpful in displacing pathogenic bacteria, allowing for their removal.
- **Creating an alkaline environment:** Cutting back on sweets, soda, tea, and coffee will reduce the acidity in the mouth. Brushing teeth with baking soda for one week may help create an alkaline environment in the mouth, making it more difficult for the pathogenic bacteria to survive.
- **Oil pulling:** Oil pulling is the Ayurvedic remedy of swishing around one tablespoon of sesame oil or coconut oil in the mouth, between the teeth, first thing in the morning for five to twenty minutes, until the oil turns white. In theory, this method helps to break down the "homes" of bacteria, which are usually made of microcapsules of oil. While water won't penetrate those microcapsules, sesame and coconut oil can, and these mix readily with the bacteria and become white in color. Then the oil is spat out along with the toxins in it.
- **Drinking cranberry juice:** Cranberry juice has been found to have anti-adhesion properties and is able to dissolve the protective coats that store the bacteria.
- **Taking oral probiotics:** Oral probiotics are an accelerated way of getting beneficial bacteria into the mouth so that they can displace pathogenic bacteria and reduce inflammation in the mouth! Dr. Jeffrey D. Hillman was able to identify strains of probiotic bacteria from volunteers with healthy teeth and gums. He isolated these bacteria and put them together in a probiotic mix called ProBiora3, which can be found in various products including EvoraPro. This type of bacterial mix works to crowd out the pathogenic bacteria and has been reported to whiten teeth, reduce gum bleeding, decrease inflammation, and reduce biofilms of pathogenic bacteria. The probiotics are available as

pretty tasty orally dissolvable mints that are to be taken twice per day for 30–90 days.

- **Using probiotic toothpaste:** Designs for Health makes PerioBiotic toothpaste, a special probiotic toothpaste that is free of fluoride and triclosan and packed with probiotics. The key to getting the most benefit from this toothpaste is to forgo rinsing your mouth after brushing your teeth, allowing the beneficial bacteria to stay in your mouth longer. It feels strange at first, but eventually you will get used to it and actually enjoy it.

ROOT CAUSE BASIC DENTAL PROTOCOL

The Root Cause Basic Dental Protocol is recommended for most people with Hashimoto's to improve their dental health, which may reduce inflammation and improve the autoimmune response.

Using xylitol, a silver-containing mouth rinse, and probiotic toothpaste three times per day over the course of six weeks can help reduce the oral pathogens in your mouth. While many cases may require the help of dental procedures and antibiotics, the following three self-care steps should help clear up pathogenic bacteria and bacterial biofilms (dental plaque) that can trigger or worsen inflammation in the mouth and lead to autoimmunity.

Step 1: Take your dental health inventory: Before you start the Root Cause Basic Dental Protocol, take a quick inventory of your mouth. Looking in the mirror, inspect your teeth before brushing and flossing. Notice and record the following:

- Receding gums
- Dark spots
- Painful teeth
- Buildup of plaque
- Loose teeth

Now, brush and floss your teeth, and note the following:

- Bleeding gums
- Pain

Keep this assessment handy, as you'll reassess and compare in six weeks.

Step 2: Follow your new dental routine:

1. Start your day with oil pulling. Swish around approximately 1 tablespoon of sesame oil or coconut oil in the mouth, between the teeth, first thing in the morning for 5–20 minutes, until the oil turns white.

2. Swish and spit with 1 teaspoon of colloidal silver liquid 3 times per day for 60 seconds. (Please note: Do not attempt to make your own colloidal silver solution. Improper preparation methods have resulted in argyria, or blue man syndrome. I recommend the following brands only: Designs for Health, Sovereign Silver, and my specially formulated Rootcology brand.)

3. Spray xylitol spray on your gums and teeth 3 times per day to help break up bacterial biofilms, or chew xylitol gum (do not chew xylitol gum with amalgam fillings, as mercury vapor is released with any kind of chewing). You can make your own xylitol spray by purchasing bulk xylitol powder (Designs for Health is one brand I like). Then use 1 teaspoon of powder in 8 oz. of fluoride-free water.

4. Use a fluoride- and triclosan-free toothpaste to brush your teeth in a jiggling motion as described previously 3 times per day.

5. Take oral probiotics 3 times per day. Garden of Life Probiotic Smile is an excellent brand. You also have the option of using a probiotic-rich toothpaste.

Step 3: Check your progress: Repeat the assessment from step 1 after doing the dental protocol for six weeks to see if you show any improvement in your oral health. If do you see an improvement, continue with your interventions and check your thyroid antibodies (if they were elevated) to see if they have decreased. Progress can be seen in antibody levels within four weeks, but the full effect of the intervention may take up to three months.

Oral care should be an ongoing effort, as plaque formation is a normal process of the mouth. However, you may be able to ease up on your dental routine after another six weeks.

Sinus Infections

Triggering infections can be present in your sinuses. These infections are often initially triggered due to yeast or mold, but they may result in a secondary bacterial infection that will also need to be treated, and it's important to be evaluated for both yeast and mold. Symptoms of sinusitis include pain in the sinuses, nose, ear, face, or throat as well as draining from the nose, headaches, chronic cough, postnasal drip, sneezing, congestion, throat irritation, loss of smell, and ear inflammation. A person may also have a fever, but that may be missed in thyroid disease.

If you have any symptoms of sinusitis, make an appointment with your ear, nose, and throat doctor to get an appropriate evaluation. The doctor may need to do a scan of your sinuses to find the infection.

To help alleviate some of the symptoms associated with sinusitis, I recommend implementing the following: a nasal rinse like the neti pot once or twice daily, the Root Cause Broad-Spectrum Gut-Cleansing Protocol, the Yeast Overgrowth Protocol, and using a silver nasal spray like Argentyn 23. To use Argentyn 23 nasal spray, administer five to ten sprays in each nostril for seven to fourteen days, then two sprays in each nostril twice per day until the infection resolves.

In some cases, more aggressive measures like antibiotics and antifungals may be necessary. Your doctor may prescribe antibiotics for your bacterial sinus infection as well as an antifungal for a fungal or yeast infection. Some people have found a special nystatin nasal flush made by compounding pharmacists to be very helpful for clearing fungal infections in the sinuses. Additionally, compounding pharmacists can also make nasal sprays that treat both fungal and bacterial infections in the nose.

A note about sinusitis: In many cases, sinusitis may be a sign that you have current or past mold exposure. If mold is your root cause, you will need to clear it out of your home (or even move if it can't be remedied) and work with a mold specialist, and you may also want to talk to your doctor about antifungal treatments. See chapter 12 for additional strategies for overcoming mold.

Epstein-Barr Virus

I suspect that many people with Hashimoto's may be suffering from a hidden Epstein-Barr infection in the thyroid gland. When I conducted a survey of 2,209 people with Hashimoto's, 11 percent of them reported that they started feeling unwell after an Epstein-Barr infection, and I know that Epstein-Barr was the virus that triggered my chronic fatigue syndrome during my freshman year in college.

A 2015 study in Poland found the virus in the thyroid cells of 80 percent of people with Hashimoto's, while controls did not have the Epstein-Barr virus in their thyroid gland. Furthermore, cells suggesting a continually proliferating state—a slowly growing infection—were found in the Hashimoto's group as well.

When a person is infected with the Epstein-Barr virus, the body's natural defense mechanisms begin to take aim at the virus. Unfortunately, in a person with poor nutrition and vulnerabilities, the virus may defeat and deplete the body's immune response, resulting in a low-grade latent infection and multiple deficiencies and imbalances that make the way for the autoimmune process to take hold.

Epstein-Barr virus has also been implicated as a trigger in many other chronic and autoimmune disorders such as multiple sclerosis, fibromyalgia, and chronic fatigue syndrome.

Epstein-Barr virus and other herpes viruses persist in their hosts for many years after the initial infection. These viruses can also become reactivated, even after many years. While I used to recommend testing for viral reactivation to begin treatment, there is emerging evidence that Epstein-Barr may still be problematic even when test results for viral reactivation are negative.

Epstein-Barr Virus Protocol

PHARMACOLOGIC TREATMENT

- Valganciclovir: 1,800 mg daily for 3 weeks, then 900 mg daily for 6 months or longer

HERBAL AND ALTERNATIVE TREATMENT

Lomatium is a broad-spectrum antiviral herb from Barlow Herbal Specialties, with potential therapeutic benefit in Epstein-Barr virus, HPV, herpes viruses, and CMV as well as for prevention of viral infections like the flu and the common cold.

Lomatium can cause a one-time rash, similar to a viral exanthem rash, that occurs as the body clears itself of a virus. To prevent the development of this rash, it is recommended to start with MunityBoost first, which is a combination of liver support herbs with a low dose of Lomatium.

If you do not use Lomatium, consider these other herbal treatments:

- Cordyceps 750 mg: 2 capsules, 3 times per day for 90 days
- Olive leaf extract: 1 capsule, 2 times per day for 60 days

SUPPORTIVE TREATMENT

- NAC: 1,800 mg per day
- ProBoost Thymic Protein A: Dr. Jacob Teitelbaum, a physician who specializes in chronic fatigue syndrome, recommends 3 packets per day for 90 days to help the body fight viruses

- Adaptogens (ashwagandha, schisandra, astragalus)
- Vitamin D: 5,000 IU per day tailored to lab testing
- Vitamin C: 500–3,000 mg per day
- Tanning in the sun or at tanning salons
- Lysine
- Intravenous vitamin C

MUNITYBOOST AND LOMATIUM CHART

Week	MunityBoost	Lomatium Dose
1	15 drops twice per day	NONE
2	25 drops twice per day	NONE
3	25 drops twice per day	25 drops twice per day
4+	NONE	25 drops twice per day

Next Steps

Tracking down an infection can often feel like trying to find a needle in a haystack. But I hope that the steps outlined in this chapter provide a clear plan of action. Successful identification and removal of an infection and its cause can have the ultimate payoff: complete healing from Hashimoto's (and the removal of other conditions and symptoms that may have developed as a result of the infection).

12

Protocols for Removing Toxins

n the Liver Support Protocol, you learned how to minimize your toxic exposure by purchasing better cleaning products, cooking utensils, personal care products, and more. But if the toxins assessment brought you here, you could have been exposed to or have ongoing exposure to a more specific toxin.

There are two main factors to consider when thinking about whether a substance can become a toxic trigger. The first, of course, is the dose of the toxin. Paracelsus, the sixteenth-century father of toxicology, said: "Poison is in everything, and no thing is without poison. The dosage makes it either a poison or a remedy." The higher the dose of the toxin, the more likely it will overburden our detoxification capabilities and make us ill. This is why reducing exposure to toxins is critical in the healing journey.

The second factor to consider is the underlying sensitivity of the exposed person. For example, in a person with celiac disease, the reaction to gluten is much greater when compared to a person with gluten sensitivity. In the former, even micro amounts of gluten can set off a severe response, while in the latter, a higher dose may be tolerated before the onset of symptoms.

While some sensitivities are genetically predetermined, there are steps we can take to make ourselves less reactive. The Fundamental Liver Support, Adrenal Recovery, and Gut Balance Protocols focused on building up your resilience to make you less sensitive and reactive to the environment around you. In some cases of toxicity, a third element must also be considered: removing the toxin from the body.

While we can reduce exposure and rebuild resilience on our own, in the case of Advanced Protocols for removing toxins from the body, you may want to work under the supervision of a qualified health care professional. This chapter will dive deeper into strategies for overcoming chemical sensitivity, electromagnetic field (EMF) sensitivity, mold, breast implant illness, heavy metal toxicity, and toxic exposure related to dental work.

Chemical Sensitivity

People with Hashimoto's are more likely to have multiple chemical sensitivities (MCS) to substances like BPA, parabens, formaldehyde, and brominated and halogenated compounds that can be found in everyday products like plastics, personal care products, furniture, and mattresses. Some symptoms of MCS include the following:

- Abnormal immune function
- Autoimmune disease
- Allergies to various substances
- Asthma-like symptoms and breathing difficulties

Reducing exposure to these chemicals is always a great idea, and the Fundamental Liver Support Protocol shared strategies like using sprouts, houseplants, and air purifiers to support our body in removing these chemicals naturally. However, people who are chemically immune reactive to one or more of these substances may need to undertake a major overhaul of their life and environment to recover their health.

Strategies for Overcoming MCS

The Cyrex Laboratories Array 11—Chemical Immune Reactivity Screen can help you determine if you are sensitive to any of nineteen

HOUSEHOLD TOXINS

Chemical	Found In	Strategy
Bisphenol A (BPA)	Plastics, receipts	Remove plastics from your cooking and food storage utensils.
Formaldehyde	Furniture made from particle board, car seats	Air out car before getting in. Avoid buying new particle board furniture.
Benzenes	In blackened food	Avoid charred, grilled, and burned foods.
Tetrachloroethylene	In dry cleaning	Opt for only "green" dry cleaning that avoids the use of these chemicals, or skip dry cleaning altogether. Air out dry-cleaned clothes before wearing.
Tetrabromobisphenol A	Flame retardants, especially in mattresses	Purchase a bromine-free mattress made of naturally flame-resistant substances like wool.
Parabens	Personal care products such as makeup, shaving cream, lotions, and shampoos	Purchase paraben-free, organic personal care products.

chemical substances. If you are found to be reactive, you may require major environmental changes to recover your health. See the Household Toxins table for guidance.

EMF Sensitivity

Another type of sensitivity that some people with Hashimoto's can have is to electromagnetic fields such as those emitted by fluorescent lights, mobile phones, Wi-Fi, cordless phones, and power lines. Symptoms of EMF sensitivity include sleep disturbances, stress, fatigue, headaches, rashes, burning sensation, pain, brain fog, and heart palpitations, any and all of which may be exacerbated with increased exposure to EMFs.

Strategies for Overcoming EMF Sensitivity

In the case of EMF sensitivity, here are some helpful strategies to feel better:

- Wire your internet access instead of using Wi-Fi.
- Do not use a laptop on your lap.
- Power off your breaker box to sleep in an electricity-free bedroom.
- Reduce or avoid the use of cell and cordless phones—opt for wired phones instead.
- Remove dimmer switches and fluorescent lights.
- Spend more time in nature!

A note about EMF sensitivity: Most of my clients who were EMF sensitive also had Lyme disease.

Mold

You may have heard of Dave Asprey, biohacker extraordinaire, the creator of Bulletproof Coffee, and the author of the *New York Times* bestselling book *The Bulletproof Diet,* but you may not know that Bulletproof Coffee and the Bulletproof Diet came out of Dave's quest to overcome Hashimoto's.

At one point, Dave weighed three hundred pounds and was constantly brain fogged and exhausted, despite eating a very low-calorie diet and exercising six days a week. He was eventually diagnosed with Hashimoto's. Dave found that gluten and toxic mold were significant triggers of his condition.

His quest to avoid toxic mold in food led him to create his signature Bulletproof Coffee—a drink low in mold and cross-reactive toxins—the Bulletproof Diet, and many supplements! Dave is now the muscular poster boy of high performance and is running a successful company, and his Hashimoto's is in remission.

In the Liver Support Protocol, I shared with you that mold can be a powerful trigger for many autoimmune conditions, including autoimmune thyroid disease, asthma, and allergies. One of the potential clues of mold being a root cause is when your health begins to deteriorate after moving into a new home.

Please note that not everyone may be affected in the same way. For example, a family member with different genes may not develop Hashimoto's but may develop asthma or allergic rhinitis soon after moving into the new home. And another family member may not have any apparent symptoms at all!

Other clues that you may be exposed to toxic mold include brain fog, breathing issues, cognitive impairment, immune suppression, fatigue, depression, arthritis, digestive problems, poor sleep, inflammation, and joint pain. Sneezing, coughing, runny nose, and asthma are the most common red flags of mold.

Testing for Mold

You can run a RealTime Laboratories test for mold metabolites in your urine to determine if mold has taken up residence in your body. Additionally, it may be helpful to do the mold panel from ALCAT lab to see which molds are reactive in your body. If you've done stool testing, sometimes the tests may reveal mold overgrowing in your gut. The mold will show up as "yeast present—taxonomy unavailable." If you suspect there may be mold in your home, you can work with a mold inspector in your area or self-order a mold test like MOLDetect.

Strategies for Overcoming Mold

You can address the presence of mold by implementing strategies in your home, following pharmacologic treatment (as prescribed by a medical professional), and taking helpful supplements. Let's look at the specifics of each of these strategies:

MINIMIZE MOLD IN YOUR HOME

- Move to a new home (easier said than done). While it's not always possible, it may become necessary.
- Work with a professional to remediate mold in your home.
- Get an air purifier for your home.
- Have the air ducts in your home cleaned.

PHARMACOLOGIC TREATMENT

- Antifungal medication like fluconazole or itraconazole: for 30–90 days for killing mold in body
- Cholestyramine powder: for 30–90 days for binding mold to carry out of the body

HERBAL AND ALTERNATIVE TREATMENT

- Oil of oregano: 2 capsules, 3 times per day for 30–60 days
- *S. boulardii:* 5 billion–15 billion CFUs, 2–4 times per day (up to 8 per day) for 60 days
- Argentyn nasal spray: 1 spray in each nostril, 1–2 times per day (for mold in sinuses)
- Activated charcoal: 2 capsules at bedtime (may cause magnesium depletion)
- CholestePure by Pure Encapsulations (soy derived): 1–2 capsules, 3 times per day (with meals) for 30–90 days

For dietary modifications: See chapter 9.

Breast Implant Illness

If you found that many of your symptoms started after breast implant surgery, you're not alone! Many of my clients have found that breast implants can be a trigger for Hashimoto's and other mystery autoimmune conditions. You may want to consider breast explant surgery to remove the implants in order to recover your health. I recommend reading the book *The Naked Truth About Breast Implants: From Harm to Healing* by Susan E. Kolb to explore your options.

Some of my readers have shared their experiences after having their breast implants removed. Here's a note from one woman who wrote to me two months after her explant surgery: "I am feeling so much better! My energy has increased greatly, I no longer have to take naps daily, and feel like I am getting myself back again. I am so excited to be able to do the house chores and run errands to more than one store and not feel exhausted from these activities any longer. I am sleeping better, no longer have memory loss or anxiety and depression. This is incredible!" Furthermore, her lab markers of TSH, thyroid antibodies, reverse T3, and inflammation showed significant improvement within weeks after removing the breast implants!

This reader's experience shows you how significant an impact breast implants can have on your health, especially as it relates to your thyroid. While this may not be true for all people, if you have Hashimoto's and breast implants, it might be worth exploring your health timeline post–implant surgery.

Toxic Metals

Numerous toxic metals have the potential to disturb thyroid function and immune system function. Humans can bioaccumulate metals, and metals have been found in the thyroid gland in biopsies. In some cases, we may be affected by one metal, in others many. We know that heavy metals can have independent, additive, and synergistic effects.

Tests for heavy metals can be ordered through functional medicine practitioners who will likely use labs such as Metametrix and Doctor's Data. These tests are usually done with a chelating agent like DMSA to pull out stored heavy metals and to determine the body's overall heavy metal burden. As shellfish can cause false positives on heavy metal tests, I recommend abstaining from shellfish for three days prior to testing.

Before attempting advanced detoxification protocols, I recommend obtaining a test of your genes, such as the one done by 23andMe, to identify any genetic mutations you may have that contribute to impaired detoxifications. Numerous genes are involved in detoxification; however, the two that I have found to be especially relevant are the MTHFR gene and the CBS gene.

If you have the MTHFR gene mutation, it's important to take N-acetylcysteine (NAC), methylfolate, and B_{12} for at least one week before a provoked urine challenge to ensure that the metals come out on the test. Hair tests can also help with analyzing toxic metal burden, but many practitioners don't know how to properly interpret hair tests, and thus positive results may be missed.

If you have come across heavy metals and heavy metal toxicity, you have probably come across chelation therapy done with chelating agents like DMSA, DMPS, and EDTA. Chelation is a therapy used to remove metals from the body. It can be very effective, but at the same time, it can be harmful, especially when done by a professional who is not fully versed in chelation (most of them are not!). Chelation can lead to toxins recirculating and taking up residence in other parts of the body, leading to other adverse reactions and even autoimmune reactions. Side effects of chelation are common, and DMSA especially can lead to a sulfur sensitivity and should not be used in those with CBS gene mutations (be sure to check for the CBS gene mutation using a test like the 23andMe before attempting chelation). Furthermore, chelation can result in depletion in important nutrients such as magnesium, molybdenum, zinc, copper, manganese, and iron. Because of the risks of chelation, I prefer to use a gentler and more polite approach to remove toxins to start (see protocols beginning on page 343).

Symptoms of toxic metal exposure vary based on the element to which you've been exposed. Here are some of the more recognizable symptoms of specific metal toxicity syndromes:

- **Nickel:** Nickel sensitivity can manifest as symptoms on the skin and within the body, such as hives, eczema, itchy skin, headaches, fatigue, and celiac-like gut symptoms. Like Hashimoto's, nickel sensitivity is a type IV hypersensitivity response. Up to 17 percent of women may be affected, and nickel sensitivity has been correlated to Hashimoto's.
- **Mercury:** Symptoms of mercury exposure include mood swings, brain fog, muscle twitching, muscle wasting, irritability, headaches, metallic taste in mouth, loss of balance, vision impairment, fatigue, and many others.
- **Arsenic:** If you've been exposed to an excess of arsenic, you might experience tingling of extremities, fatigue, hair loss, depression, darkening of skin, weakness, muscle wasting, and cough.
- **Copper:** Symptoms of toxicity include fatigue, irritability, anxiety, emotional lability, hair turning orange, acne, poor concentration, skin rashes, and poor wound healing.
- **Lead:** Lead toxicity symptoms might manifest as muscle weakness, fatigue or lethargy, ADHD, irritability, myalgia, joint pain or arthritis, loss of appetite, unusual taste, headache, insomnia, decreased libido, weight loss, personality changes, neurological challenges, neuropathy, nausea, vomiting, memory loss, depression, and incoordination.

Strategies for Overcoming Metal Toxicity

Rather than forcefully pushing out heavy metals, I like to usher them out gently and politely by reducing exposure, using competitive nutrients to our advantage, and incorporating sauna therapy, especially infrared sauna, which can be very helpful in healing. We'll look at these strategies as well as an overall Gentle Metal Detoxification Protocol first. Then I'll go into specific protocols for sulfur and copper.

Reduce Exposure

As I've mentioned before, the key to reducing your exposure to any element or substance is knowing where to find it. You can use this chart to help reduce exposure to nickel, lead, arsenic, mercury, and cadmium and help your body clear them.

Boost Competitive Nutrients

One of the keys to clearing out toxins and even preventing them from binding receptors within our bodies is to keep those receptors occupied with nutrients and minerals. This is why I recommend multiple vitamins and minerals to prevent the toxins from binding within our bodies. Some especially useful vitamins and minerals are selenium, zinc, molybdenum, iodine, and B vitamins.

It's also important to make sure you have sufficient levels of glutathione, an important molecule that detoxifies heavy metals. I've already recommended NAC and selenium methionine, which boost your glutathione levels, but you can also take oral liposomal glutathione to increase levels.

Sauna Therapy

Sauna therapy can help to increase our internal body temperature, giving our thyroid a much-needed break from trying to increase it for us. Saunas have shown benefit in chronic fatigue syndrome, pain, and fibromyalgia. Using a sauna one to five times per week over the course of one to three months is the schedule that has been most frequently studied.

Most of my clients with Hashimoto's really love sauna therapy and report that it makes them feel cozy, happy, and relaxed as it gives them more energy. However, sauna therapy is not for everyone; if you're drinking alcohol or are hungover, please avoid the sauna, as this combination

METAL TOXICITY SOURCES

Metal	Food Sources	Environmental Sources	Practices to Aid Clearance
Nickel	Chocolate, nuts, canned foods, black tea, shellfish, processed meats with fillings or casings, beans, lentils, soy, peas, wheat, oatmeal, buckwheat, seeds, bean sprouts, Brussels sprouts, asparagus, broccoli, cauliflower, spinach, canned vegetables	Stainless steel cookware and utensils, vitamins with nickel, tap water	Take vitamin C with each meal, eat a high-iron diet, take a zinc supplement, and replace stainless steel cookware. Sweat!
Lead	Rice from China, wild game shot with lead bullets, wine	Indoor dust, cosmetics (such as lipsticks), gasoline, crystals, toys from China, lead pipes	Take vitamin D, exercise, and eat greens.
Arsenic	Rice, chicken, shellfish	Well water, lipsticks, insecticides, copper-treated wood, Ayurvedic supplements	Take turmeric, NAC, and chlorophyll. Take methylation support supplements like those used for the MTHFR gene mutation.

Metal	Food Sources	Environmental Sources	Practices to Aid Clearance
Mercury	Certain fish, especially king mackerel, marlin, orange roughy, shark, swordfish, tilefish, ahi tuna, and bigeye tuna	Coal-burning plants, amalgams, vaccines	Alkalize the urine with a magnesium or potassium supplement to boost clearance. Take a selenium supplement.
Cadmium	Shellfish, organ meat	Cigarette smoke, pesticide spray, air	Alkalize the urine with a magnesium or potassium supplement to boost clearance. Sweat!

can lead to a dangerous electrolyte imbalance. Reported sauna-related adverse events are rare, but people with heart conditions, diabetes, and other chronic conditions should check with their doctors before proceeding. Here are some other tips for a great sauna session:

- Stay hydrated. You're going to be sweating quite a bit, so it's easy to get dehydrated. I recommend drinking purified water so you know you're not putting toxins back in through water.
- If you feel light-headed or unwell, get out.
- Begin with short segments of time in the sauna and then gradually stay longer as your body adjusts and can handle it better.

Gentle Metal Detoxification Protocol

Two important parts of detoxification involve mobilizing the toxins and adsorbing the toxins. Mobilizing toxins can be done with prescription chelating agents or cilantro in concentrated form. As I often find that people with Hashimoto's report feeling worse rather than better after prescription chelation agents, I prefer to use cilantro to start.

The second important part of detoxification is adsorbing the toxins so they stick to the substance and are ushered to removal rather than roaming free within the body. Various substances are used for adsorbing toxins, such as chlorella, activated charcoal, and fiber as apple pectin or psyllium. I personally have preferred activated charcoal and psyllium husk fiber, as chlorella can be problematic for some with Hashimoto's due to high iodine content and immune-modulating properties associated with seaweeds.

The following is a gentle protocol for heavy metals. The duration of treatment will depend on the toxic load.

- A psyllium mixture can help adsorb toxins from the gut and prevent their reabsorption by stimulating bile excretion. Psyllium has the added benefit of lowering cholesterol and blood sugar, preventing gallstone formation, and increasing colonic butyrate, which boosts good bacteria. Charcoal and psyllium should be used together, as psyllium can prevent charcoal-induced constipation. Add 1 teaspoon of psyllium husks to 8 oz. of water and mix. Drink mixture, and then follow with one more 8 oz. cup of water. Be sure to separate from food and other supplements by 2 hours. Utilize this mixture 1–3 times per day.
- Activated charcoal can help clear toxins from the intestinal tract and appendix and prevents hepatic recycling of toxins. Start with 1 capsule of activated charcoal daily apart from meals (midday around 3:00 to 4:00 P.M. usually works best for most people), and then work your way up to 3 capsules. Be sure to supplement with magnesium citrate, as activated charcoal can deplete magnesium and lead to constipation and other symptoms of magnesium deficiency.
- Cilantro mobilizes toxins. Take 2 drops twice per day before meals (or 30 minutes after charcoal or psyllium mixture) for 1

week on, then 3 weeks off. May repeat for 1 week each month to move toxins out gradually and gently.

- Apple pectin or rice bran fiber may also be used as sources of fiber that can help with clearing out toxins from the body. Take 7 to 10 g per day.
- Alpha-lipoic acid is a sulfur-containing supplement that can help reduce heavy metals and increase glutathione levels. Take 100 to 300 mg per day. (Avoid with CBS gene mutation.)

A note about fiber: Ideally, you will have cleared out any gut infections, especially SIBO, as you're working on detoxification. Detoxification protocols that contain fiber can aggravate SIBO, dysbiosis, and other types of gut imbalances.

If you do have toxins in your body, it may also help to continue taking vitamin C, a multivitamin, betaine with pepsin (heavy metals deplete stomach acid), probiotics, magnesium, zinc, selenium, and NAC as you work on clearing them out of your body. Furthermore, you may also want to repeat the Fundamental Liver Support Protocol while detoxifying.

It may also be helpful to ensure that your urine is alkaline, which can increase the elimination of toxins. A urine pH above 7 is recommended. If you find that your urine pH continues to be lower (or more acidic), you can try supplementing with magnesium to enhance alkalization. You can find pH sticks online to measure the pH of your urine.

Sulfur Sensitivity

I have found that individuals with the CBS gene mutation are more likely to have sulfur sensitivity. Sulfur requires specific protocols to encourage elimination. In some cases, sulfur toxicity or sensitivity may be present in people with mercury toxicity, and some of my clients have reported this reaction after treatment with DMSA. Symptoms of sulfur toxicity include skin rashes and reactions to sulfur-rich foods such as eggs and garlic.

SULFUR TOXICITY PROTOCOL

- Follow a 2-week vegan diet cleanse (if tolerated).
- Avoid sulfur-rich foods such as eggs, garlic, onions, and cruciferous vegetables for 4–8 weeks.
- Supplement with butyrate, molybdenum, B_{12}, L-carnitine, and thiamine to help to clear out excess sulfur for 4–8 weeks.
- Avoid sulfur-containing supplements, including NAC, selenium, glutathione, and alpha-lipoic acid for 4–8 weeks.

Copper Toxicity

Copper toxicity is a relatively common root cause for Hashimoto's. Symptoms include fatigue, irritability, anxiety, emotional lability, hair turning reddish, acne, poor concentration, skin rashes, and poor wound healing.

You might have been exposed to excess copper through water coming through old copper pipes, food, multivitamins, birth control pills, copper IUDs, and some dental procedures. Copper toxicity can also be a result of poor adrenal function or excess estrogen.

These are ways to test for copper toxicity:

- **Hair test:** Elevated copper may show up directly or be hidden, where the copper looks normal but results show high calcium and low zinc-to-copper ratio, or high calcium and high mercury.
- **Blood test:** Copper toxicity may show up as low alkaline phosphatase.
- **Genova Diagnostics Comprehensive Urine Element Profile provoked with DMPS/DMSA:** This test will show elevations in copper.

Supporting the adrenals, balancing female hormones, taking supplements, and following a low-copper diet can be helpful in eliminating copper toxicity.

COPPER DETOX DIET

Yes Foods High in Zinc, Low in Copper	No Foods High in Copper
Eggs	Organ meats like liver
Poultry	Shellfish
Wild game	Shrimp
Red meat	Lobster
Fish	Crab
Vegetables	Oysters*
Ginger	Plant proteins (beans, peas, soy)
Cinnamon	Nuts
Filtered water	Seeds
	Mushrooms
Occasional (once a week)	Chocolate*
Pumpkin seeds	Avocados
Legumes	Brewer's yeast
Gluten-free grains	Curry
	Black pepper
	Black tea
	Beer

*Very high levels of copper

COPPER TOXICITY PROTOCOL (LISTED IN ORDER OF IMPORTANCE)

Please note, the duration of treatment will depend on the overall copper load.

- Copper-free multivitamin (Nutrient 950 from Pure Encapsulations): 6 per day
- Zinc picolinate: 30–60 mg per day to displace copper
- Molybdenum: 100–500 mcg per day to clear out copper from bloodstream
- Manganese: 5–30 mg per day to displace copper
- Vitamin C: 500–3,000 mg per day to chelate copper
- B_6: 50–200 mg per day to aid with symptoms of copper toxicity

- Alpha-lipoic acid: 50–150 mg per day to chelate copper
- Evening primrose oil: 500 mg twice per day to improve zinc absorption

Copper Dumps

It's important to note that copper protocols may result in mild worsening of symptoms during the first ten days of treatment. Then improvements will be noticeable in weeks three to four, and full effects may be seen in three to twelve months. Within the first couple of days, you might experience copper dumps, which can occur as you begin to clear copper in large quantities. These can include symptoms of nausea, racing thoughts, anxiety, irritability, emotional volatility, and skin flare-ups.

To read more about overcoming copper toxicity, I highly recommend checking out the excellent book *Why Am I Always So Tired?* by Ann Louise Gittleman.

As copper toxicity often co-occurs with adrenal dysfunction, continuing fish oils, NAC, magnesium, B complex, and adrenal support may also be wise if you have copper toxicity. Additionally, adding higher doses of evening primrose oil (2,000 to 3,000 mg per day) can help with symptoms including hair loss.

MTHFR Gene Variation

In the Liver Support Protocol, I introduced you to the MTHFR gene variation, which may complicate some of the protocols used to help those with Hashimoto's. The MTHFR gene mutation causes a potential impairment in methylation, which is one of the body's main ways of getting rid of heavy metals, and individuals who have this mutation may have a propensity for impaired clearance of heavy metals.

The MTHFR gene variation can lead to elevated homocysteine levels, which can in turn create nutrient deficiencies in folate, B_6, and B_{12}. Individuals with the MTHFR gene variation may also have a difficult time processing folic acid (a manufactured version of folate) that is present in low-quality supplements and added to processed foods.

In addition to lifestyle changes, individuals with the MTHFR gene variation and high levels of homocysteine may benefit from activated versions of folate, B_6, and B_{12} such as in methylfolate (also known as L-5-MTHF), pyridoxal-5'-phosphate (P5P), and methylcobalamin, respectively. This is because we may not be able to get enough of the needed nutrients from food alone. The Rootcology Methylation Support, Pure Encapsulations Homocysteine Factors, and Designs for Health Homocysteine Supreme are supplements that contain all of the above-mentioned ingredients and may be helpful for supporting methylation in those with the MTHFR gene mutation.

Testing for homocysteine and the MTHFR gene variation is available through many labs. 23andMe offers a test for the MTHFR gene, and many individuals can get the tests from their physicians covered by insurance.

Many of the lifestyle interventions helpful for Hashimoto's are also helpful for the MTHFR gene variation. It's important to note that not everyone with Hashimoto's has this variation. A recent study by Arakawa and colleagues of thyroid patients with Hashimoto's and Graves' found that polymorphisms were as common in autoimmune thyroid disease as they were in the normal population.

MTHFR GENE SUPPLEMENT PROTOCOL

I also recommend adding betaine with pepsin (for extra trimethylglycine) and Nutrient 950 from Pure Encapsulations as a multivitamin.

MTHFR MUTATION PROTOCOL

Rootcology Methylation Support, Pure Encapsulations Homocysteine Factors, and Designs for Health Homocysteine Supreme are MTHFR support supplements with activated B_6 (as pyridoxal-5-phosphate), activated folate, and B_{12} as methylcobalamin and trimethylglycine.

Homocysteine Test Results	Number of Capsules per Day
<6 µmol/L	1
6–9 µmol/L	2
9–15 µmol/L	3
>15 µmol/L	5

Dental Work

Another important part of minimizing your toxin exposure could include evaluating dental procedures you've had over the years, which could have exposed you to certain heavy metals and radiation. As part of the Advanced Protocols for removing toxins, I recommend that you consider any dental work you've had and how it might have played a role in your thyroid symptoms. Let's take a deeper look at some of the possible sources of exposure and strategies for addressing them.

Dental Amalgams

Did you know that if you have dental amalgam fillings, also called silver fillings, you actually have mercury in your mouth? In fact, amalgams contain 50 percent mercury by weight. They also contain small amounts of silver, tin, copper, and zinc. Amalgams are a major source of mercury exposure in the general population, accounting for two-thirds of human mercury exposure. Mercury is continuously released from the fillings every time a person chews, as mercury vapor is not a chemically stable compound. Rates of absorbed mercury from amalgam fillings range from 9 to 17 mcg/d, with an uptake estimate of 12 mcg/d.

A 2006 forensic study found that mercury from amalgams does accumulate in thyroid tissue. In the study, the more mercury fillings a person had, the higher amount of mercury was deposited in their thyroid gland. Additionally, the same study found that mercury also concentrates in the brain, pituitary gland, and kidneys. Another study found that babies of women with amalgam fillings may also have mercury deposits in their organs and experience an impact on thyroid function. The higher the maternal levels of mercury in the blood, the higher the TSH levels in the children.

Collected research has revealed links between mercury exposure and autoimmunity. Here are some of the research highlights:

- Case reports of accidental mercury ingestion have demonstrated that mercury may trigger an autoimmune response in some individuals.
- Mercury also has well-documented endocrine activity and has been found to cause excess T4 levels and depress the concentrations of biologically active T3 in animals.
- Mercury can deplete the body of selenium and the antioxidants that require selenium. Selenium deficiency, as well as a deficiency in antioxidants, has been recognized as a Hashimoto's trigger.
- In 2010, Hybenova and colleagues reported that some individuals may present with a delayed hypersensitivity to nickel or mercury. This type of reaction can be measured with the commercially available lymphocyte transformation test, LTT-MELISA.
- In 2006, thirty-nine patients with Hashimoto's thyroiditis were tested with the MELISA test for hypersensitivity to inorganic mercury. The patients with mercury hypersensitivity who underwent amalgam replacement showed a significant decrease in the levels of both anti-TG and anti-TPO antibodies.
- Another report utilizing the MELISA test in a few autoimmune diseases found that replacement of amalgam fillings

with composite fillings in mercury-allergic subjects resulted in improvement of health in about 70 percent of patients. Several laboratory parameters, such as mercury-specific lymphocyte responses in vitro and antithyroid antibodies, were normalized as well.

Based on this research, if you are someone with Hashimoto's and amalgam fillings, I encourage you to take the MELISA test. The test can be obtained from a biological dentist who has an account with the laboratory that offers the test. This test will help you determine whether removing your fillings should be a priority at this time or if other interventions may be more important.

If you determine that you need to have your amalgams removed, it's important to have it done safely. If the removal is not done properly, the removal process can actually cause you to breathe in additional mercury vapor. Instead of a low dose of mercury over time, you will get the big dose of mercury all at once. If you have the MTHFR gene mutation and intestinal permeability, all that mercury can overburden your detox pathways.

Many of my clients have reported an onset or increase in Hashimoto's symptoms after improper amalgam removal. Ask your dentist for the following precautions for safe removal of dental amalgams:

- The dentist should use a rubber dam.
- You should receive an oxygen mask and skin cover.
- Extra suction should be in place to evacuate the vapors away from you.
- After the procedure, be sure to rinse your mouth with activated charcoal, which can bind up residues.

Ideally, I would also recommend that you go through the Liver Support Protocol and the Gut Balance Protocol before you attempt to have your amalgam fillings replaced. This will give your detox capabilities extra support. Some dentists will also have you take NAC or another liver support supplement before, during, and after your amalgam removal.

If you have had amalgam fillings replaced without taking the proper precautions, I would again recommend that you go through the Liver Support and Gut Balance Protocols and then work with your doctor to test for residual heavy metals through a heavy metal–provoked urine challenge to determine if you need additional medical interventions.

Dental X-Rays

Even small amounts of radiation have been found to be of detriment to the thyroid gland, so it's wise to limit your exposure to radiation. Digital x-rays are safer than film x-rays and provide less radiation. I would also highly recommend that you use a thyroid shield or guard. Unfortunately, some dental assistants may only give you a chest guard. Don't let them pressure you into doing the x-rays without properly protecting your thyroid gland! You can also purchase your own thyroid guard to bring to appointments with you.

Biocompatible Dental Materials

Fillings, onlays, bridges, braces, plastic aligners (like Invisalign), and other types of materials used for dental work may trigger an immune response in some individuals.

It may not be necessary or feasible to remove these materials in most cases (with the exception of Invisalign, which is easily removable). For future dental work, however, I would encourage anyone with an autoimmune condition and their family members to start working with a biological dentist to be tested for biocompatibility. We are all unique and may react to different materials, so it will be up to your biological dentist to help you determine the safest materials for your unique biochemistry when it's time to get a new filling or replace an old one (reports for the life of composite fillings vary from seven to twenty years after the filling is placed).

Testing to determine if you are sensitive to the chemical and materials in your dental work can be done through a biological dentist who works with Clifford Materials Reactivity Testing.

Next Steps

I hope that this chapter helped you remove and recover from toxic triggers, and that this process has both eliminated your symptoms and produced intense feelings of relief. I know for myself and many of my clients, this has been the case—nothing feels quite as good as getting rid of something that's doing you harm and stealing your health!

Author's Note

It is my sincere hope that this book will serve you on your journey in recovering your health!

For many of you, the protocols in this book will produce a complete health transformation—you will be free to live your life with energy, vitality, passions, and purpose, and your symptoms will soon become a distant memory! For others, this book may be just the starting point that helps you take back your health in the days and years to come.

Wherever you are on your journey, I want you to remember that you are not alone and that you have the power to take back your health. There are many paths to healing, and I hope my guidance has helped you find your own way.

I'm honored to have been a part of your journey, and I hope that we can stay connected. My passion for helping people with Hashimoto's grows deeper with every new discovery, with every success story, and with every client challenge that leads me to seek more solutions.

I love to connect with readers to learn about the successes and challenges they have had, and I love to share the latest and greatest developments in overcoming Hashimoto's. Let's stay in touch! You can find me on social media and by visiting my website. I hope to see you there!

To your continued health,
Izabella Wentz, PharmD, FASCP
www.thyroidpharmacist.com
www.facebook.com/thyroidlifestyle

Gratitude

'd like to thank the following people who have helped me get this book out of my brain and onto the bookshelves so that it could transform countless lives:

Michael Wentz, my sweet hubby—for your unwavering love and support, for walking by my side, for holding my hand on this journey! I love dreaming with you, growing with you, and blazing our own trail. I know that as long as we have each other, anything is possible.

Marta Nowosadzka, my beautiful and brilliant mother, who inspired me to be a healer and continues to inspire me each day—for always believing in me and supporting me, for being the best mama and role model a girl could ever ask for! Adam Nowosadzki, my warm and clever dad—for nurturing my empathy and compassion, for always understanding my sensitive soul, for showing me that I can blaze my own trail. Robert Nowosadzki, my favorite brother—for showing me that I can create my own destiny, for always having my back! Amanda Nowosadzki, my soul sister—for being a blossom of kindness, love, and inspiration! The whole Wentz family—for the love and acceptance that you've given me!

Brittany, Katie, Anna, Claudia, Heather, and the rest of my Root Cause Advocates behind the curtains—for holding down the fort, allowing me to focus on doing what I do best! I'm so lucky to have a team that genuinely cares about the work that we do in the world.

Alan Christianson—for your friendship and encouragement, for taking a little pharmacist under your wing. Collaborating with you has been a dream come true! Andrea Nakayama, my dear Hashi sister—for your big-sisterly encouragement, friendship, and advice in my growing journey. Magdalena Wszelaki, my Polish Hashi sister—for your friendship, the delicious food, and our deep conversations! I'm eternally grateful for your coaching on the beach in San Diego! JJ Virgin—for being such a generous mentor and guide! Donna Gates—for believing in me and for saying that sometimes it's the petite women with soft voices who change the world! Datis Kharrazian—for your encouragement of my work. It has meant the world to me!

My Root Cause Rebel friends: Steve Wright, Leanne Ely, Mickey Trescott, Hashimoto's Awareness, ThyroidChange, Hashimoto's 411, Dana Trentini, Marc Ryan, Eric Osansky, Shannon Garrett, Kirk Gair, Michelle Corey, Mary Shomon, James Maskell, Dave Asprey, Katie Wells, Mark Hyman, Kelly Brogan, Suzy Cohen, Sean Croxton, Danna Bowman, Christa Orecchio, Aviva Romm, Peter Osborne, Trudy Scott, Jolene Brighten, Michael Roesslein, David Brady, Tom O'Bryan, Melanie and James Roche, and many others—for the change we're creating together!

The gifted healers I've met along the way, especially Elena Koles, David Luce, and Katherine Ward—for helping me on my journey.

My publishing dream team: Celeste Fine and John Maas, my awesome literary agents—for giving me a chance to shine, for your faith in me, for your support in every step of the publishing process. I feel like I won the agent lottery with you two! The rock stars at Harper One, especially Gideon Weil and Gretchen Lees—for partnering with me to create this book and shaping it to make it as approachable and helpful as possible! Courtney Kenney—for your wonderful ideas and project management prowess!

My clients and readers—for your curiosity and commitment to healing. I'm so proud of you for taking charge of your own health, and I'm grateful to be a part of your healing journeys! My wonderful reader, Tereska Wankowicz, for asking me for a protocol-based book.

Selected Bibliography

In order to maximize the amount of helpful information in this book and due to publisher-driven book-length constraints, I chose to bring you more content, which required limiting the references provided within this book. I've selected key references to list here. You'll find the complete, extensive bibliography of up-to-date references, for free, at www.thyroid pharmacist.com/action, should you wish to review the scientific evidence for this book.

Ajjan, R., and A. Weetman. 2015. "The pathogenesis of Hashimoto's thyroiditis: Further developments in our understanding." *Hormone and Metabolic Research* 47 (10): 702–10. doi:10.1055/s-0035–1548832.

Arena, S., A. Latina, R. Baratta, G. Burgio, D. Gullo, and S. Benvenga. 2015. "Chronic lymphocytic thyroiditis: Could it be influenced by a petrochemical complex? Data from a cytological study in South-Eastern Sicily." *European Journal of Endocrinology* 172 (4): 383–89. doi:10.1530/eje-14–0864.

Bajaj, J., P. Salwan, and S. Salwan. 2016. "Various possible toxicants involved in thyroid dysfunction: A review." *Journal of Clinical and Diagnostic Research* 10 (1): FE01–3. doi:10.7860/jcdr/2016/15195.7092.

Baldini, M., A. Colasanti, A. Orsatti, et al. 2009. "Neuropsychological functions and metabolic aspects in subclinical hypothyroidism: The effects of l-thyroxine." *Progress in Neuropsychopharmacology and Biological Psychiatry* 33 (5): 854–59. doi:10.1016/j .pnpbp.2009.04.009.

Bellis, M., L. Burke, P. Trickett, and F. Putnam. 1996. "Antinuclear antibodies and thyroid function in sexually abused girls." *Journal of Traumatic Stress* 9 (2): 369–78. doi:10.1007/bf02110669.

Bertalot, G., G. Montresor, M. Tampieri, et al. 2004. "Decrease in thyroid autoantibodies after eradication of *Helicobacter pylori* infection." *Clinical Endocrinology* 61 (5): 650–52. doi:10.1111/j.1365–2265.2004.02137.x.

Bozkurt, N., B. Karbek, E. Cakal, H. Firat, M. Ozbek, and T. Delibasi. 2012. "The association between severity of obstructive sleep apnea and prevalence of Hashimoto's thyroiditis." *Endocrine Journal* 59 (11): 981–88. doi:10.1507/endocrj.ej12–0106.

Bunevicius, A., J. Leserman, and S. Girdler. 2012. "Hypothalamicpituitary-thyroid axis function in women with a menstrually related mood disorder." *Psychosomatic Medicine* 74 (8): 810–16. doi:10.1097/psy.0b013e31826c3397.

Carta, M., A. Loviselli, M. Hardoy, et al. 2004. "The link between thyroid autoimmunity (antithyroid peroxidase autoantibodies) with anxiety and mood disorders in the community: A field of interest for public health in the future." *BMC Psychiatry* 4 (1). doi:10.1186/1471-244x-4-25.

Contis, G., and T. Foley. 2015. "Depression, suicide ideation, and thyroid tumors among Ukrainian adolescents exposed as children to Chernobyl radiation." *Journal of Clinical Medicine Research* 7 (5): 332–38. doi:10.14740/jocmr2018w.

Costantini, A., and M. I. Pala. 2014. "Thiamine and Hashimoto's thyroiditis: A report of three cases." *Journal of Alternative and Complementary Medicine* 20 (3): 208–11. doi:10.1089/acm.2012.0612.

Daher, R. 2009. "Consequences of dysthyroidism on the digestive tract and viscera." *World Journal of Gastroenterology* 15 (23): 2834. doi:10.3748/wjg.15.2834.

Davies, T. 2016. "Pathogenesis of Hashimoto's thyroiditis (chronic autoimmune thyroiditis)." *Uptodate.com.* Accessed August 30, 2016. http://www.uptodate.com/contents/pathogenesis-of-hashimotos-thyroiditis-chronic-autoimmune-thyroiditis.

Drutel, A., F. Archambeaud, and P. Caron. 2013. "Selenium and the thyroid gland: More good news for clinicians." *Clinical Endocrinology* 78 (2): 155–64. doi:10.1111/cen.12066.

Duntas, L. 2009. "Autoimmunity: Does celiac disease trigger autoimmune thyroiditis?" *Nature Reviews Endocrinology* 5 (4): 190–91. doi:10.1038/nrendo.2009.46.

Eglite, M., T. Zvagule, K. Rainsford, J. Reste, E. Čurbakova, and N. Kurjane. 2009. "Clinical aspects of the health disturbances in Chernobyl nuclear power plant accident clean-up workers (liquidators) from Latvia." *Inflammopharmacology* 17 (3): 163–69. doi:10.1007/s10787-009-0001-4.

Farahid, O., N. Khawaja, M. Shennak, et al. 2014. "Prevalence of coeliac disease among adult patients with autoimmune hypothyroidism in Jordan." *Eastern Mediterranean Health Journal* 20 (1): 51–55.

Fasano, A. 2011. "Zonulin and its regulation of intestinal barrier function: The biological door to inflammation, autoimmunity, and cancer." *Physiological Reviews* 91 (1): 151–75. doi:10.1152/physrev.00003.2008.

———. 2012. "Leaky gut and autoimmune diseases." *Clinical Reviews in Allergy & Immunology* 42 (1): 71–78. doi:10.1007/s12016-011-8291-x.

Friedman, M., S. Wang, J. Jalowiec, G. McHugo, and A. McDonagh-Coyle. 2005. "Thyroid hormone alterations among women with posttraumatic stress disorder due to childhood sexual abuse." *Biological Psychiatry* 57 (10): 1186–92. doi:10.1016/j.biopsych.2005.01.019.

Galletti, P., and G. Joyet. 1958. "Effect of fluorine on thyroidal iodine metabolism in hyperthyroidism." *Journal of Clinical Endocrinology & Metabolism* 18 (10): 1102–10. doi:10.1210/jcem-18-10-1102.

Garber, J., R. Cobin, H. Gharib, et al. 2012. "Clinical practice guidelines for hypothyroidism in adults: Cosponsored by the American Association of Clinical Endocrinologists and the American Thyroid Association." *Thyroid* 22 (12): 1200–1235. doi:10.1089/thy.2012.0205.

Gartner, R. 2002. "Selenium supplementation in patients with autoimmune thyroiditis decreases thyroid peroxidase antibodies concentrations." *Journal of Clinical Endocrinology & Metabolism* 87 (4): 1687–91. doi:10.1210/jc.87.4.1687.

Gierach, M., J. Gierach, A. Skowrońska, et al. 2012. "Hashimoto's thyroiditis and carbohydrate metabolism disorders in patients hospitalised in the Department of Endocrinology and Diabetology of Ludwik Rydygier Collegium Medicum in Bydgoszcz between 2001 and 2010." *Endokrynologia Polska* 63 (1): 14–17.

Hadithi, M. 2007. "Coeliac disease in Dutch patients with Hashimoto's thyroiditis and vice versa." *World Journal of Gastroenterology* 13 (11): 1715. doi:10.3748/wjg.v13.i11.1715.

Haviland, M., J. Sonne, D. Anderson, et al. 2006. "Thyroid hormone levels and psychological symptoms in sexually abused adolescent girls." *Child Abuse & Neglect* 30 (6): 589–98. doi:10.1016/j.chiabu.2005.11.011.

Heckl, S., C. Reiners, A. Buck, A. Schäfer, A. Dick, and M. Scheurlen. 2015. "Evidence of impaired carbohydrate assimilation in euthyroid patients with Hashimoto's thyroiditis." *European Journal of Clinical Nutrition* 70 (2): 222–28. doi:10.1038/ejcn.2015.167.

Hoang, T., C. Olsen, V. Mai, P. Clyde, and M. Shakir. 2013. "Desiccated thyroid extract compared with levothyroxine in the treatment of hypothyroidism: A randomized, double-blind, crossover study." *Journal of Clinical Endocrinology & Metabolism* 98 (5): 1982–90. doi:10.1210/jc.2012–4107.

Höfling, D., M. Chavantes, M. Acencio, et al. 2014. "Effects of low-level laser therapy on the serum TGF-⊠1 concentrations in individuals with autoimmune thyroiditis." *Photomedicine and Laser Surgery* 32 (8): 444–49. doi:10.1089/pho.2014.3716.

Höfling, D., M. Chavantes, A. Juliano, et al. 2010. "Low-level laser therapy in chronic autoimmune thyroiditis: A pilot study." *Lasers in Surgery and Medicine* 42 (6): 589–96. doi:10.1002/lsm.20941.

Hybenova, M., P. Hrda, J. Procházková, V. Stejskal, and I. Sterzl. 2010. "The role of environmental factors in autoimmune thyroiditis." *Neuroendocrinology Letters* 31 (3): 283–89.

Jack, A., A. Dawson, K. Begany, et al. 2013. "fMRI reveals reciprocal inhibition between social and physical cognitive domains." *NeuroImage* 66:385–401. doi:10.1016/j.neuroimage.2012.10.061.

Janegova, A., P. Janega, B. Rychly, K. Kuracinova, and P. Babal. 2015. "The role of Epstein-Barr virus infection in the development of autoimmune thyroid diseases." *Endokrynologia Polska* 66 (2): 132–36. doi:10.5603/EP.2015.0020.

Joung J., Y. Cho, S. Park, et al. 2014. "Effect of iodine restriction on thyroid function in subclinical hypothyroid patients in an iodine-replete area: A long period observation in a large-scale cohort." *Thyroid* 24 (9): 1361–68. doi:10.1089/thy.2014.0046.

Juby, A., M. Hanly, and D. Lukaczer. 2016. "Clinical challenges in thyroid disease: Time for a new approach?" *Maturitas* 87:72–78. doi:10.1016/j.maturitas.2016.02.001.

Katarzyna, K., C. Jarosz, S. Agnieszka, et al. 2013. "L-thyroxine stabilizes autoimmune inflammatory process in euthyroid nongoitrous children with Hashimoto's thyroiditis and type 1 diabetes mellitus." *Journal of Clinical Research in Pediatric Endocrinology* 5 (4): 240–44. doi:10.4274/jcrpe.1136.

Kogelnik, A., K. Loomis, M. Hoegh-Petersen, F. Rosso, C. Hischier, and J. Montoya. 2006. "Use of valganciclovir in patients with elevated antibody titers against human herpesvirus-6 (HHV-6) and Epstein-Barr virus (EBV) who were experiencing central nervous system dysfunction including long-standing fatigue." *Journal of Clinical Virology* 37:S33–S38. doi:10.1016/s1386–6532(06)70009–9.

Kvantchakhadze, R. 2002. "Wobenzym in the complex treatment of autoimmune thyroiditis." *International Journal of Immunorehabilitation* 4 (1): 114.

Lauritano, E., A. Bilotta, M. Gabrielli, et al. 2007. "Association between hypothyroidism and small intestinal bacterial overgrowth." *Journal of Clinical Endocrinology & Metabolism* 92 (11): 4180–84. doi:10.1210/jc.2007-0606.

Luiz, H., D. Gonçalves, T. Silva, et al. 2014. "IgG4-related Hashimoto's thyroiditis: A new variant of a well known disease." *Arquivos Brasileiros de Endocrinologia & Metabologia* 58 (8): 862–68. doi:10.1590/0004-2730000003283.

Mansournia, N., M. Mansournia, S. Saeedi, and J. Dehghan. 2014. "The association between serum 25OHD levels and hypothyroid Hashimoto's thyroiditis." *Journal of Endocrinological Investigation* 37 (5): 473–76. doi:10.1007/s40618-014-0064-y.

Mariani, M., A. Palpacelli, A. Mussoni, and A. Rossodivita. 2013. "Hashimoto's thyroiditis: An accidental discovery of a lingual thyroid in a 7-year-old child." *BMJ Case Reports*, August 21. doi:10.1136/bcr-2013-200247.

Mehrdad, M., F. Mansour-Ghanaei, F. Mohammadi, F. Joukar, S. Dodangeh, and R. Mansour-Ghanaei. 2012. "Frequency of celiac disease in patients with hypothyroidism." *Journal of Thyroid Research* 2012:1–6. doi:10.1155/2012/201538.

Messina, G., T. Esposito, J. Lobaccaro, et al. 016. "Effects of low-carbohydrate diet therapy in overweight subject with autoimmune thyroiditis: Possible synergism with ChREBP." *Drug Design, Development and Therapy* 214 (10): 2939–46. doi:10.2147/dddt.s106440.

Moncayo, R., and H. Moncayo. 2015a. "Proof of concept of the WOMED model of benign thyroid disease: Restitution of thyroid morphology after correction of physical and psychological stressors and magnesium supplementation." *BBA Clinical* 3:113–22. doi:10.1016/j.bbacli.2014.12.005.

———. 2015b. "The WOMED model of benign thyroid disease: Acquired magnesium deficiency due to physical and psychological stressors relates to dysfunction of oxidative phosphorylation." *BBA Clinical* 3:44–64. doi:10.1016/j.bbacli.2014.11.002.

Müssig, K., A. Künle, A. Säuberlich, et al. 2012. "Thyroid peroxidase antibody positivity is associated with symptomatic distress in patients with Hashimoto's thyroiditis." *Brain, Behavior, and Immunity* 26 (4): 559–63. doi:10.1016/j.bbi.2012.01.006.

Naiyer, A., J. Shah, L. Hernandez, et al. 2008. "Tissue transglutaminase antibodies in individuals with celiac disease bind to thyroid follicles and extracellular matrix and may contribute to thyroid dysfunction." *Thyroid* 18 (11): 1171–78. doi:10.1089/thy.2008.0110.

Nanan, R., and J. Wall. 2010. "Remission of Hashimoto's thyroiditis in a twelve-year-old girl with thyroid changes documented by ultrasonography." *Thyroid* 20 (10): 1187–90. doi:10.1089/thy.2010.0102.

Nexo, M., T. Watt, B. Cleal, et al. 2014. "Exploring the experiences of people with hypo-and hyperthyroidism." *Qualitative Health Research* 25 (7): 945–53. doi:10.1177/1049732314554093.

Pacini, F., T. Vorontsova, E. Molinaro, et al. 1998. "Prevalence of thyroid autoantibodies in children and adolescents from Belarus exposed to the Chernobyl radioactive fallout." *Lancet* 352 (9130): 763–66. doi:10.1016/s0140-6736(97)11397-6.

Patil, B., and G. Giri. 2012. "A clinical case report of Hashimoto's thyroiditis and its impact on the treatment of chronic periodontitis." *Nigerian Journal of Clinical Practice* 15 (1): 112. doi:10.4103/1119-3077.94113.

Patil, B., T. Gururaj, and S. Patil. 2011. "Probable autoimmune causal relationship between periodontitis and Hashimoto's thyroiditis: A systemic review." *Nigerian Journal of Clinical Practice* 14 (3): 253. doi:10.4103/1119-3077.86763.

Peckham, S., D. Lowery, and S. Spencer. 2015. "Are fluoride levels in drinking water associated with hypothyroidism prevalence in England? A large observational study of GP practice data and fluoride levels in drinking water." *Journal of Epidemiology & Community Health* 69 (7): 619–24. doi:10.1136/jech-2014-204971.

Plaza, A., L. Garcia-Esteve, C. Ascaso, et al. 2010. "Childhood sexual abuse and hypothalamus-pituitary-thyroid axis in postpartum major depression." *Journal of Affective Disorders* 122 (1–2): 159–63. doi:10.1016/j.jad.2009.07.021.

Popławska-Kita, A., M. Kościuszko-Zdrodowska, K. Siewko, et al. 2015. "High serum IgG4 concentrations in patients with Hashimoto's thyroiditis." *International Journal of Endocrinology* 2015:1–6. doi:10.1155/2015/706843.

Prummel, M., and W. Wiersinga. 2005. "Thyroid peroxidase autoantibodies in euthyroid subjects." *Best Practice & Research Clinical Endocrinology & Metabolism* 19 (1): 1–15. doi:10.1016/j.beem.2004.11.003.

Rajič, B., J. Arapović, K. Raguž, M. Bošković, S. Babić, and S. Maslać. 2015. "Eradication of *Blastocystis hominis* prevents the development of symptomatic Hashimoto's thyroiditis: A case report." *Journal of Infection in Developing Countries* 9 (7): 788–91. doi:10.3855/jidc.4851.

Rotondi, M., L. de Martinis, F. Coperchini, et al. 2014. "Serum negative autoimmune thyroiditis displays a milder clinical picture compared with classic Hashimoto's thyroiditis." *European Journal of Endocrinology* 171 (1): 31–36. doi:10.1530/eje-14-0147.

Sategna-Guidetti, C. 2001. "Prevalence of thyroid disorders in untreated adult celiac disease patients and effect of gluten withdrawal: An Italian multicenter study." *American Journal of Gastroenterology* 96 (3): 751–57. doi:10.1016/s0002-9270(00)02410-2.

Staii, A., S. Mirocha, K. Todorova-Koteva, S. Glinberg, and J. Jaume. 2010. "Hashimoto thyroiditis is more frequent than expected when diagnosed by cytology which uncovers a pre-clinical state." *Thyroid Research* 3 (1): 11. doi:10.1186/1756-6614-3-11.

Sterzl, I., J. Procházková, and P. Hrda. 2006. "Removal of dental amalgam decreases anti-TPO and anti-Tg autoantibodies in patients with autoimmune thyroiditis." *Neuroendocrinology Letters* 27, suppl. 1: 25–30.

Strieder, T. 2008. "Prediction of progression to overt hypothyroidism or hyperthyroidism in female relatives of patients with autoimmune thyroid disease using the Thyroid Events Amsterdam (THEA) score." *Archives of Internal Medicine* 168 (15): 1657. doi:10.1001/archinte.168.15.1657.

Sugiyama, A., H. Nishie, S. Takeuchi, M. Yoshinari, and M. Furue. 2015. "Hashimoto's disease is a frequent comorbidity and an exacerbating factor of chronic spontaneous urticaria." *Allergologia et Immunopathologia* 43 (3): 249–53. doi:10.1016/j.aller.2014.02.007.

Şükran, D., B. Ömer, Ş. Damla Gökşen, and Ö. Samim. 2011. "Clinical course of Hashimoto's thyroiditis and effects of levothyroxine therapy on the clinical course of the disease in children and adolescents." *Journal of Clinical Research in Pediatric Endocrinology* 3 (4): 192–97. doi:10.4274/jcrpe.425.

Toulis, K., A. Anastasilakis, T. Tzellos, D. Goulis, and D. Kouvelas. 2010. "Selenium supplementation in the treatment of Hashimoto's thyroiditis: A systematic review and a meta-analysis." *Thyroid* 20 (10): 1163–73. doi:10.1089/thy.2009.0351.

Vojdani, A., and I. Tarash. 2013. "Cross-reaction between gliadin and different food and tissue antigens." *Food and Nutrition Sciences* 4 (1): 20–32. doi:10.4236/fns.2013.41005.

Vykhovanets, E., V. Chernyshov, I. Slukvin, et al. 1997. "131I dose-dependent thyroid autoimmune disorders in children living around Chernobyl." *Clinical Immunology and Immunopathology* 84 (3): 251–59. doi:10.1006/clin.1997.4379.

Wang, J., S. Lv, G. Chen, et al. 2015. "Meta-analysis of the association between vitamin D and autoimmune thyroid disease." *Nutrients* 7 (4): 2485–98. doi:10.3390 /nu7042485.

Wentz, I. 2015. "Top 9 takeaways from 2232 people with Hashimoto's." *Thyroid Pharmacist.* Accessed August 30, 2016. http://www.thyroidpharmacist.com/blog /top-10-takeaways-from-2232-people-with-hashimotos.

Wentz, I., and M. Nowosadzka. 2013. *Hashimoto's Thyroiditis.* Lexington, KY: Wentz, LLC.

Xu, J., X. Liu, X. Yang, et al. 2011. "Supplemental selenium alleviates the toxic effects of excessive iodine on thyroid." *Biological Trace Element Research* 141 (1–3): 110–18. doi:10.1007/s12011-010-8728-8.

Yang, S. 2010. "Exposure to flame retardants linked to changes in thyroid hormones." *Berkeley News,* June 21. Accessed October 19, 2016. http://news.berkeley .edu/2010/06/21/pbde/.

Index

adaptogenic herbs, 181–82
Addison's disease, 155, 156
adrenal glands: additional resources on, 305; adrenal fatigue, 151–53, 154–57; adrenal glandulars, 305; Adrenal Recovery Protocol for, 37, 69–70, 81, 147–89, 219; Advanced Adrenal Support Protocol for, 300–305; all about the, 150–53; hormones and testing the, 88, 151–53, 156, 302–4; supplements supporting, 188–89
Adrenal Recovery Protocol (four weeks): Adrenal Assessment, 148–49; adrenal supplement overview, 188–89; five steps of the, 149, 163–87; next steps and roadblocks, 188; overview of the, 37, 69–70, 81, 147–48, 162, 219
Adrenal Recovery Protocol steps: 1: rest, 149, 164–66; 2: de-stress, 149, 166–70; 3: reduce inflammation, 149, 170–72; 4: balance the blood sugar, 150, 172–80; 5: replenish nutrients and add adaptogens, 150, 181–87
Advanced Adrenal Support Protocol, 300–305
Advanced Protocols: Addressing Infections, 73, 312–20; Advanced Adrenal Support Protocol, 300–305; Copper Toxicity Protocol, 346–47; defining role of triggers in, 222–23; description and focus of, 66, 70, 72, 76; Epstein-Barr Virus Protocol, 329–30; gut infections and recommended, 312–20; Mastering Nutrition and Nutrients, 72; MTHFR Gene Supplement Protocol, 348–49; Optimizing Thyroid Hormones, 72; Overcoming Traumatic Stress, 72–73; periodontitis and protocols, 321–25; Removing Toxins, 73; Resetting Your Stress Response, 291–300; Root Cause Basic

Dental Protocol, 325–27; Root Cause Broad-Spectrum Gut-Cleansing Protocol, 320, 327; two ways to approach the, 224; Yeast Overgrowth Protocol, 317, 327. *See also* detoxification; Fundamental Protocols; Hashimoto's Protocol; Root Cause Assessments
alcohol, 116, 129–30
allergies: food, 101, 262–63; as symptoms of Hashimoto's, 17, 18, 19, 43
anti-inflammatory environment, 284–85
anxiety, 186
Armour Thyroid, 35, 237–39, 243
aromatherapy, 255–56
assessments. *See* Root Cause Assessments
autoimmune conditions: autoimmune-emotion connection, 292–93; celiac disease co-occurrence with, 103–4; co-occurrence of other, 48, 50–51; debunking hygiene hypothesis on, 308; other types of, 48; theories on development of, 49–50; three factors present in development of, 5, 7, 46–49
autoimmune thyroid disorders: conventional medical model for treating, 2–3; co-occurrence of other autoimmune conditions, 48, 50–51; how they develop, 46–48; three factors for, 5, 7, 46–49. *See also* Hashimoto's thyroiditis
Ayurvedic medicines toxicity, 138

Blastocystis hominis, 311, 315–16
blood sugar: balanced, 150, 172–80; habits to stabilize, 177–78; imbalanced, 157, 160–62; stressors of and how food impacts your, 175–80
brain fog/memory loss, 17
breast implant illness, 337
broad-spectrum gut infection, 319–20

B$_{12}$ Deficiency Overview, 281
B$_{12}$ vitamin, 136, 137, 181, 184, 189, 216, 280–81
B vitamins (B$_2$, B$_3$, B$_5$, B$_6$, B$_{12}$), 136–37, 181, 182–85, 189

caffeine: avoiding, 111, 114–15, 118, 135, 165–66, 174, 270; health effects of, 71, 105, 107, 108, 109
Candida genus, 316
carbohydrate intake, 161, 175, 264
CBS gene, 338
celiac disease: co-occurrence with autoimmune disorders, 103–4; gluten-containing foods and, 102–6, 108, 109; testing for, 109–10
chemical sensitivity, 332, 334
Chernobyl radiation exposure, 96, 101
chronic inflammation, 157, 162
compounded thyroid medications, 24, 35, 237–39, 243
conventional medicine: autoimmune thyroid disorders treatment by, 2–3; medication bias of, 240–41; searching for lifestyle intervention alternative to, 23–26. *See also* doctors; thyroid medications
copper detox diet, 346
copper toxicity, 345
Copper Toxicity Protocol, 346–47
cosmetics, 96–99
cruciferous veggies, 120, 121–22, 130
cytology test, 55, 56
Cytomel, 237, 239, 243

dehydroepiandrosterone (DHEA), 24
dental health: biocompatible dental materials, 352–53; dental amalgams, 349–52; dental x-rays, 352; periodontitis, 321–25; Root Cause Basic Dental Protocol, 325–27. *See also* health
detoxification: reducing toxic exposure strategies, 110, 132–35; support detox pathways strategies, 44. *See also* Advanced Protocols; Fundamental Protocols
diagnosis: additional food sensitivity

testing, 261–63; author's experience with getting a, 3–5, 15–26; empathy vs. logic and grieving your, 30–31; getting a definitive, 51–52; importance of early, 59. *See also* laboratory testing
dietary modifications: additional modifications for specific symptoms, 274–76; carbohydrate intake, 264; iodine intake, 266, 267–69; real food smoothies, 265–66; Root Cause Rotation Diet, 266, 270–73
diets: copper detox, 346; dangerous diet dogmas, 259–61; low-carbohydrate, 161; note on infections and, 319; Root Cause Autoimmune Diet, 200–201, 262; Root Cause Paleo Diet, 171–72, 262; Root Cause Rotation Diet, 266, 270–73. *See also* nutrition
DIG-AT-IT approach: *Hashimoto's Protocol* for using the, 9–11; identifying Hashimoto's triggers using, 5
digestive enzymes, 201–4
dining out suggestions, 117
doctors: doctor shopping, 19–20, 31; finding Dr. Right, 34–37; functional medicine practitioners, 35–37; second-opinion resources, 244. *See also* conventional medicine; thyroid medications
dogmas: as barrier to health, 31, 74; dangerous diet, 259–61

Easy Bone Broth, 209–10
EMDR (eye movement desensitization and reprocessing) therapy, 298, 300
EMF sensitivity, 334
empathy vs. logic, 30–31
environmental factors, 47–48
enzymes: deficiencies, 196–98; digestive, 201–4; proteolytic, 204–6
epigenetics, 47
Epstein-Barr virus, 312, 328–29
Epstein-Barr Virus Protocol, 329–30
essential oils, 255–56
exercise recommendations, 166–69, 174

fats, 176–77
fermented foods, 206

ferritin (iron), 216, 278–80
fight-or-flight mode, 152, 287
fluoride, 94–95, 133
food allergies, 101, 262–63
food pharmacology: food sensitivities
    and food allergies, 101–6; under-
    standing food toxins through, 100
foods: dining out suggestions, 117;
    fermented, 206; Food and Hunger
    Guide, 176; Food Reintroduction
    Chart, 278; impacts on your blood
    sugar, 175–77; list of supportive,
    110, 116–32; reactive, 196–98,
    200–201, 278; remove potentially
    triggering, 110, 111–16; Root Cause
    Rotation Diet excluded and in-
    cluded, 270–73. See also meal plans;
    nutrition
food sensitivities: common food reac-
    tions and symptoms, 106–9; food
    allergies compared to, 101; Food
    Reintroduction Chart to watch for,
    278; gluten-containing foods and,
    102–6, 108, 109; Hashimoto's and,
    102–9; testing for celiac disease and,
    109–10, 261–63
free T3, 57, 244–46
free T4, 57, 244–46
functional medicine practitioners, 35–37
Fundamental Protocols: Adrenal
    Recovery Protocol, 37, 69–70, 81,
    147–89, 219; as central to your health
    plan, 71–72; description and focus of
    the, 66, 69, 76, 80–81; Gut Balance
    Protocol, 37–38, 71, 81–82, 191–220;
    Liver Support Protocol, 37, 44, 69,
    81, 83–145, 219. See also Advanced
    Protocols; detoxification

genetic triggers: CBS gene, 338; DIG-
    AT-IT approach to identifying, 5;
    MTHFR gene mutation, 136, 138,
    139, 140, 142, 143, 202, 282, 338,
    347–49; predisposition as autoimmu-
    nity factor, 3, 7, 47–49
glutamine, 210
gluten sensitivity: to gluten-containing
    foods, 102–6, 108, 109, 111; non-

celiac gluten sensitivity (NCGS),
    104; testing for, 109–10
Green Juice, 123
Gut Balance Protocol (six weeks): four
    steps of the, 196–215; Gut Health
    Assessment, 195–96; Gut-Health
    Supplement Overview, 217–18;
    next steps and roadblocks, 215–17;
    overview of the, 37–38, 70, 81–82,
    191–94, 219–20
Gut Balance Protocol steps: 1: remove
    reactive foods, 196, 200–201; 2: sup-
    plement with enzymes, 196, 201–6;
    3: balance the gut flora, 196, 206–9;
    4: nourish the gut, 196, 209–15
gut infections and protocols: Blastocystis
    hominis, 311, 315–16; broad-spectrum
    gut infection, 319–20; H. pylori,
    311, 313–14; note on diets for, 319;
    overview of, 312–13; SIBO, 311–12,
    317–19; yeast overgrowth, 311,
    316–17. See also infections

hair loss, 8, 19, 42, 78
Hashimoto's Protocol: Adrenal Recovery
    Protocol (four weeks), 37, 69–70, 81,
    147–89, 219; Gut Balance Proto-
    col (six weeks), 37–38, 71, 81–82,
    191–220; Liver Support Protocol (two
    weeks), 37, 44, 69, 81, 83–145, 219;
    overview of the, 9–11, 37–38, 65. See
    also Advanced Protocols; treatments
Hashimoto's thyroiditis: at-risk popu-
    lations, 3; author's experience with,
    3–5, 15–26; description of and
    increasing rate of, 1; development
    and three triggers of, 5, 7, 46–49; five
    stages of, 57–59; as underlying cause
    of hypothyroidism, 1, 2. See also auto-
    immune thyroid disorders; remission
Hashimoto's Thyroiditis: Lifestyle Interven-
    tions for Finding and Treating the Root
    Cause (Wentz), 4, 9, 24, 26, 73–74,
    266, 269
health: achieving the dream of, 76,
    78–80; making time for yourself
    to improve, 28–30; sometimes the
    patient knows best about their, 22;

health (*continued*)
taking charge of your own, 26, 28.
See also dental health
health plan: creating your, 63; Fundamental Protocols as central to your,
71–72. *See also* remission
health team members, 77–78
hives (chronic spontaneous urticaria), 51
household toxins, 333
HPA axis (hypothalamic-pituitary-
adrenal axis), 151–53
HPA axis malfunction, 154–55, 157
H. pylori, 311, 313–14
hyperthyroidism, 42
hypothyroidism, 1, 2, 42

IADC (induced after-death communication), 298
immune system: how Hashimoto's
affects the, 1; IgG, IgA, and IgM
branches of the, 262–63
infections: Advanced Protocols for
addressing, 73, 312–20; Epstein-Barr
virus, 312, 328–30; Infections Assessment, 226–27; linked to Hashimoto's,
309–11; note on diets for, 319; sinus,
327–28; testing for, 311–12; as a
trigger, 66, 67. *See also* gut infections
and protocols
inflammation reduction, 163, 170–72
intestinal permeability. *See* leaky gut
(intestinal permeability)
iodine intake, 266, 267–69
Iron Deficiency Overview, 280

laboratory testing: ACTH test and
blood cortisol levels, 156, 302–4;
celiac disease and food sensitivities,
109–10, 261–63; copper toxicity, 345;
cytology, 55, 56; ferritin, vitamin
D, vitamin B₁₂, 216; free T3 and
free T4, 57, 244–46; fundamental
nutrient testing, 278–82; for mold,
335–36; recommended, 35–36;
SIBO, 319; for specific infections,
311–12; thyroid ultrasound, 55–56;
TPO antibodies and TG antibodies, 54–55, 56, 249, 250; TSH

(thyroid-stimulating hormone), 24,
52–54, 58, 59, 233, 236, 242, 244,
245–47; 21-hydroxylase autoantibody
test, 156. *See also* diagnosis
leaky gut (intestinal prmeability): description of the, 47, 48, 88, 191–94;
Gut Balance Protocol to heal the,
37–38, 70, 81–82, 191–218, 219–20
levothyroxine (Synthroid), 3, 21–22, 23,
58, 60, 237, 239, 243
lifestyle interventions: author's search for,
23–26; to complement conventional
treatment, 23–26, 60–61; epigenetics
findings on importance of, 47; finding
purpose in life, 27–28; *Hashimoto's
Thyroiditis* on one-off interventions,
24; making time for yourself, 28–30
liothyronine (T3), 237, 239, 240–
41, 243
lip gloss toxicity, 97–98
liver detoxification: cautions regarding
forceful, 87–89; harm of too early, 89;
support pathways to, 110, 135–45
liver dysfunction: Liver Assessment,
84–86, 145; understanding causes of,
83–84
Liver Support Protocol (two weeks): additional interventions and protocols to
support, 145; cautions regarding use of,
87–90; four steps of the, 110–45; how
it works, 110–11; overview of the, 37,
44, 69, 81, 86–87, 219; understanding
the reasons behind the, 83–84
Liver Support Protocol meal plans:
breakfasts and snacks, 126–28,
130–31; dinners, 132; liver support
recipes, 128–30; lunches, 131–32;
Sample Daily Meal Plan, 131
Liver Support Protocol steps: 1: remove
potentially triggering foods, 110,
111–16; 2: add supportive foods, 110,
116–32; 3: reduce toxic exposure,
110, 132–35; 4: support detox pathways, 110, 135–45
logic vs. empathy, 30–31
low-dose naltrexone (LDN), 251–52
low-level laser therapy (LLLT), 252–54

magnesium: need for, 187; supplements
for, 141–42, 144, 189
meal plans: Liver Support Protocol,
126–32; Root Cause Rotation Diet,
273. See also foods
medications. See thyroid medications
mental and emotional stress, 157,
159–60
metal toxicity: copper, 345–47; overview
and sources of, 337–39, 341–42;
strategies for overcoming, 339–40,
342–44
Modified Root Cause Build Smoothie,
265–66
mold: exposure to, 92–93, 334–35; testing and treatments for, 335–36
MTHFR gene mutation: description and
cautions on, 136, 138, 139, 140, 142,
143, 202, 282, 338; MTHFR Gene
Supplement Protocol, 348–49
multiple chemical sensitivities (MCS),
332, 334

N-acetylcysteine (NAC), 212, 218
natural desiccated thyroid medications
(NDTs), 35, 237–39, 240–41, 243
Nature-Throid, 35, 237–39, 240, 243
nonprescription thyroid glandulars,
254–55
nutrients: adrenal supplements, 181–89;
Advanced Protocols for mastering,
72; B₁₂ Deficiency Overview, 281;
gut-health supplements, 209–15,
217–18; Iron Deficiency Overview,
280; liver support supplements,
136–45; replenish, 150, 181–87;
suggestions for mastering, 276–77;
symptoms indicating need for, 276–
77; testing for, 278–82; transferring
to nutrient-dense plan, 126
nutrition: Advanced Protocols for mastering, 72; Nutrition Assessment, 225.
See also diets; foods

omega-3 fatty acids, 212–13, 218

periodontitis: description of, 321; treatments for, 321–25

personal care products toxicity, 96–99
Pilates and yoga, 167–68, 174
polycystic ovary syndrome (PCOS), 78
positive thinking, 169
probiotics, 207–9, 217
protein: poorly digested proteins, 196–
98; sources and intake of, 176–79
proteolytic enzymes, 204–6
Protocol for Resetting Your Stress
Response steps: 1: practice self-love
and self-kindness, 294–95; 2: develop
attitude of gratitude, 295–96; 3: seek
alpha brain waves, 296; 4: find support in community, 296; 5: be willing
to seek deeper treatments, 298, 300
PTSD (post-traumatic stress disorder),
291, 298
purpose in life, 27–28

radiation exposure, 96, 101
reactive foods: description of, 196–98,
200–201; Food Reintroduction Chart
to watch for, 278
remission: author's experience with diagnosis and, 3–5, 15–26; DIG-AT-IT
approach identifying triggers, 5;
overview of the journey toward, 6–8;
personal behaviors that can impact,
31–32. See also Hashimoto's thyroiditis; health plan
rest (Adrenal Recovery Protocol), 163,
164–66. See also sleep apnea
Root Cause Approach: guidelines for
success using the, 73–76; health benefits of the, 8; preparing to use the,
65–66, 68–69
Root Cause Assessments: Adrenal Assessment, 148–49; Gut Health Assessment, 195–96; Infections Assessment,
226–27; Liver Assessment, 84–86,
145; Nutrition Assessment, 225; Thyroid Hormones Assessment, 224–25;
Thyroid Symptom Assessment,
62; Toxins Assessment, 227–28;
Traumatic Stress Assessment, 226;
Undertreatment or Overtreatment
Assessment, 248. See also Advanced
Protocols; symptoms

Root Cause Autoimmune Diet,
200–201, 262
Root Cause Basic Dental Protocol,
325–27
Root Cause Broad-Spectrum
Gut-Cleansing Protocol, 320, 327
Root Cause Build Smoothie, 178
Root Cause Green Smoothie, 118–20
Root Cause Paleo Diet, 171–72, 262
Root Cause Rebels: author's community
of, 5, 10; becoming a, 32–34; food sensitivities among the, 106–9; on what it
feels like to have Hashimoto's, 45–46
Root Cause Reflections: changing the
voice inside your head, 299–300; getting ready for action, 38–39; Hashimoto's anxiety, 186; a journey through
trauma, 301; reporting on possible
triggers in life, 67–68; sometimes the
patient knows best, 22; what it feels
like to have Hashimoto's, 45–46; what
makes you feel better?, 164
Root Cause Research Corner: Addison's
disease, 156; autoimmune theories,
49–50; debunking hygiene hypothesis, 308; fluoride conspiracy, 95;
iodine controversy, 267–69; obstructive sleep apnea (OSA) and Hashimoto's, 158; Root Cause Medication
Survey, 239; Root Cause TSH Survey,
247; social stress, 297; stevia, 180;
thiamine, 185
Root Cause Rotation Diet: foods to
exclude and include, 270–73; meal
ideas, 273; overview of the, 266, 270
Root Cause Smoothie, 127, 177

selenium, 185, 187, 189
SIBO, 311–12, 317–19
sick building syndrome, 91–92
sinus infections, 327–28
sleep apnea, 157–59. See also rest (Adrenal Recovery Protocol)
smoothies: Modified Root Cause Build
Smoothie, 265–66; Root Cause
Build Smoothie, 178; Root Cause
Green Smoothie, 118–20; Root Cause
Smoothie, 127, 177

stevia, 180
stress. See traumatic stress
success stories: behavioral barriers to,
31–32; behaviors leading to, 32; Root
Cause guidelines for, 73–76
sulfur sensitivity, 344–45
supplements: adrenal supplements,
181–89; caution about toxins in
Ayurvedic medicines, 138; gut-
health supplements, 209–15, 217–18;
liver support supplements, 136–45;
methylation-support, 139
surgical treatment, 61
symptoms: commonly described
Hashimoto's, 2, 8, 16–20; dietary
modifications for specific, 274–76;
food sensitivities, 106–9; of hypothyroidism and hyperthyroidism, 42, 43;
indicating need for nutrients, 276–77;
remission as no manifestation of, 7;
unique to Hashimoto's, 43–44. See
also Root Cause Assessments
Synthroid (levothyroxine), 3, 21–22, 23,
58, 60, 237, 239, 243

T3 (triiodothyronine), 57, 58, 110
T3 medications (liothyronine), 237, 239,
240–41, 243
T4 (thyroxine), 57, 58, 110
T4 medications (levothyroxine), 3,
21–22, 23, 58, 60, 237, 243
T4/T3 combination medications,
237–39, 243
Tandoori Chicken, 125
TG antibodies (thyroglobulin antibodies), 54–55, 56, 205
thiamine, 185
thyroid antibodies: range for person without disease, 7; TPO antibodies and TG
antibodies, 54–55, 56, 205, 249, 250
thyroid gland: description of the, 41–42;
Hashimoto's autoimmune destruction
of the, 1
thyroid hormones: Advanced Protocols
for optimizing, 72; hyperthyroidism
as overabundance of, 42; hypothyroidism as deficiency of, 2, 42;
produced by thyroid gland, 41–42;

T1, T2, T3, T4, and calcitonin, 57, 58, 110
Thyroid Hormones Assessment, 224–25
thyroid medications: caution about overdosing, 247–48; final thoughts on optimizing, 256–57; the four Rs of optimal use of, 232–40, 242, 244–46; liothyronine (T3), 237, 239, 240–41, 343; natural desiccated thyroid medications (NDTs), 35, 237–39, 240–41, 243; regaining thyroid function therapies and, 248–56; Root Cause Medication Survey, 239; summary of, 243; Synthroid (levothyroxine) [T4], 3, 21–22, 23, 58, 60, 237, 239, 343; T4/T3 compounded thyroid medications, 24, 35, 237–39, 243; weaning, 256. *See also* conventional medicine; doctors; treatments
thyroid medications Four Rs: 1: Right Person: are you a candidate?, 232–34; 2: Right Way: are you taking medications to ensure proper absorption?, 234–36; 3: Right Drugs: are you on the right type?, 236–41; 4: Right Dose: are you taking the right amount?, 242, 244–46
Thyroid Pharmacist blog, 77
Thyroid Symptom Assessment, 62
thyroid ultrasound, 55–56
toxic exposure: cleaning products, 99; cooking utensils, 100; copper, 345–47; dental amalgams, 349–52; everyday life, 93–95; fluoride, 94–95; food pharmacology on sensitivities and allergies, 100–110; metal toxicity, 337–47; mold, 92–93, 334–36; personal care products, 96–99; radiation, 96; reduce your, 110, 132–35; sick building syndrome, 91–92; sulfur sensitivity and, 344–45; Toxins Assessment, 227–28
toxic load: autoimmune disease and higher, 88; cautions for liver detoxification to reduce, 87–89
toxins: acceptable vs. harmful, 68; Advanced Protocols for removing,

73; Hashimoto's trigger category of, 66, 90–110; household, 333; multiple chemical sensitivities (MCS), 332, 334; in supplements, 138
TPO antibodies (thyroid peroxidase antibodies), 54–55, 56, 205, 249, 250
traumatic stress: blood sugar imbalances, 157, 160–62; chronic inflammation, 157, 162; creating anti-inflammatory environment to reduce, 284–85; feeling unsafe and, 287–89; Hashimoto's and, 285–86; HPA axis response to, 152–53; inadequate sleep, 157–59; mental and emotional, 157, 159–60; overcoming traumatic events and patterns, 286, 290–91; Protocol for Resetting Your Stress Response, 291–300; PTSD (post-traumatic stress disorder), 291, 298; social stress form of, 297; Traumatic Stress Assessment, 226
Traumatic Stress Assessment, 226
treatments: considering surgery as, 61; lifestyle interventions to complement medication, 23–26, 60–61. *See also* Hashimoto's Protocol; thyroid medications
TRH (thyrotropin-releasing hormone), 250
triggers: being aware of your, 66, 68; defining and their role in Advanced Protocols, 222–23; DIG-AT-IT approach to identifying, 5; genetic, 7, 47–49; infection category of, 66, 67; reflecting on your, 67–68; toxin category of, 66, 68, 90–110
TSH (thyroid-stimulating hormone): description and levels of, 24, 52–54, 58, 59, 233, 236, 242, 244, 245–47; Root Cause TSH Survey, 247
turmeric tea, 124–25
twin studies, 47–48

Undertreatment or Overtreatment Assessment, 248

vertigo, 51
vitamin B₁₂, 136, 137, 181, 184, 189, 216, 280–81

vitamin C, 137, 185, 189, 279
vitamin D, 213–15, 216, 218
vitamins A, D, E, K, 137
vitamins B (B$_2$, B$_3$, B$_5$, B$_6$, B$_{12}$), 136–37,
    181, 182–85, 189
vulnerabilities: description of, 65–66;
    overcoming triggers by fixing, 68–69

water: bottled, 133; fluoride in the,

94–95, 133; green your, 133–34
Way of the Wounded Healer, 27–28
WP Thyroid, 35, 237–39, 240, 243

yeast overgrowth, 311, 316–17
Yeast Overgrowth Protocol, 317, 327
yoga and Pilates, 167–68, 174

zinc, 210–12, 218